Prenatal Testosterone in Mind

Prenatal Testosterone in Mind
Amniotic Fluid Studies

Simon Baron-Cohen
Svetlana Lutchmaya
Rebecca Knickmeyer

A Bradford Book
The MIT Press
Cambridge, Massachusetts
London, England

First MIT Press paperback edition, 2006

© 2004 Massachusetts Institute of Technology

Set in Sabon by The MIT Press.

Library of Congress Cataloging-in-Publication Data

Baron-Cohen, Simon.
Prenatal testosterone in mind : amniotic fluid studies / Simon Baron-Cohen, Svetlana Lutchmaya, Rebecca Knickmeyer.
p. cm.
"A Bradford book."
Includes bibliographical references and index.
ISBN 978-0-262-02563-8 (hc), 978-0-262-52456-8 (pb)
1. Amniotic liquid—Analysis. 2. Fetus—Growth. 3. Testosterone.
I. Lutchmaya, Svetlana. II. Knickmeyer, Rebecca. III. Title.

RG627.B37 2004
155.4—dc22   2003069132

Contents

Preface

This is a book about a scientific journey. In our lab, we have been doing something a little bit different. We have not shared it with the outside world until now.

We have written this book primarily for our colleagues in cognitive neuroscience. We do not pretend that it is anything other than technical, specialized, and for the reader with a good background in biology. The general reader may get the gist, but this is a book aimed specifically at our colleagues who have never considered investigating testosterone and who might, after reading about our journey, consider including measures of this vital chemical in their own work. For the general reader, there are other books that are far more accessible; one is *The Essential Difference* (Baron-Cohen 2003).

If you were to visit our lab, you would at first glance think it was just an ordinary set of offices full of graduate students and research associates. But a few minutes later you would in all likelihood notice the enormous deep freezer in Rebecca and Svetlana's office. What lies in the freezer is quite enticing, at least to us. There are thousands of little test tubes, each filled with amniotic fluid from a mother in the Cambridgeshire vicinity. Each test tube represents a child, the vast majority of who are now happy and healthy 4-year-olds running around Cambridge.

Our research question, which we have pursued doggedly these last 5 years, is this: What, if any, is the relationship between the level of fetal testosterone in the test tube and the child's behavior at the ages of 1, 2, and 4 years?

Each of these test tubes turns out to be—we think—science's best way of getting at a lost past: namely, what was going on chemically when a particular child was in the womb. This isn't about Freudian speculations about the woman on the couch in front of you and whether her early years shaped her adult outcome. Yes, we are interested in the developmental precursors and—dare we say it?—causes of later cognition and behavior. But the test tubes of amniotic fluid mean that we no longer have to be prone to all the potential errors of retrospective speculation or retrospective measurement. We can study development prospectively, from week 16 of gestation, and we can make predictions about the future brain, mind, and behavior of a little fetus.

What could be more exciting to a scientist?

Before you jump on board with us, we should discuss the ethical issues. Amniotic fluid doesn't just fall into scientists' laps. The only reason we scientists even have this opportunity to study neurocognitive development prospectively in this way is that a woman decided, or was advised, to undergo amniocentesis.

In and of itself, amniocentesis is now quite a routine obstetric procedure. Most pregnant women over the age of 35 are encouraged to undergo it, since the risk of having a child with Down's Syndrome increases with age. This is where the ethical issues associated with our research begin. Leaving aside the ethical decision the woman made in opting to have an "amnio," would she also opt for termination of her pregnancy if markers of Down's Syndrome were identified in the fluid? The fact of the matter is that at the point of "donating" her amniotic fluid to the hospital she was not giving consent for it to be the subject of our research.

"Amnios" are almost invariably stressful. A long needle is needed to draw fluid from the womb, and the expert doctor doing it uses the latest ultrasound technology to ensure that the needle does not touch the fetus. But even so, it is known that a small percentage of pregnancies end in miscarriage after amniocentesis. Thankfully, 98 percent of "amniocentesized" fetuses go on to develop normally and healthily.

The first important ethical step toward using amniotic fluid for scientific study other than that for which it was intended is to obtain fresh consent from each mother. In this book, in addition to explaining the biological interest and the technical issues, and in addition to describing the exciting results obtained from such studies, we detail the ethical issues so that others who are considering similar studies can appreciate how delicate, sensitive, and important this aspect of the work is.

It was crucial to ensure that we would not ask a mother for consent to reanalyze her amniotic fluid (perhaps stored for years) if her pregnancy had sadly ended with a miscarriage or a stillbirth, or if she had opted for termination. To keep a potentially distressing letter from being sent to one of these women inappropriately, Svetlana and Rebecca, the pioneering doctoral students who embarked on the studies described in this book, spent hundreds if not thousands of hours systematically going through the medical records of each and every one of the women. The strategy was approved by each hospital's Ethics Committee.

Some may object to the term "amniocentesized children." We could not think of another term that so precisely describes who we are studying, and we wanted to put these children at center stage in the play you are about to witness. We hope you will appreciate that these are not children with any medical condition, despite the clinical sound of the term. They are ordinary, happy, healthy, naughty, fun-loving, lovable children who just happen to be a bit different from other children in one respect: their mothers opted for amniocentesis. That may mean the children are not exactly representative of the general population, in that their mothers may be a bit older than average. But from the scientific perspective, we think they are very special. They give us a window—almost like a fossil record—into life in the womb, with which we can compare their current behavior.

Although this book is aimed at our colleagues in cognitive neuroscience, we feel that we are acting as intermediaries between endocrinology and psychology. These two fields are not complete strangers; there is a long tradition of studying the effects of hormones on behavior. The novelty of our work lies in our focus on fetal hormones and their effects on postnatal behavior.

We hope you enjoy the discoveries described in these pages. We still find it remarkable that a few drops of testosterone can affect how much eye contact a toddler makes, or the size of a toddler's vocabulary. These results are counterintuitive. It is widely believed that behaviors such as eye contact and language must be determined by the social environment (parents, sibs, peers) rather than the biological environment. But the statistics say otherwise. True, the social world makes a contribution, but, as this book shows, so does biology.

Peter Raggatt and Kevin Taylor, biochemists at Addenbrooke's Hospital, guided our investigations and encouraged us to pursue them in the face of what at times seemed like a mountain of practical obstacles. Gerald Hackett, an obstetrician at the Rosie Maternity Hospital, and Steve Smith, head of that hospital, backed our study and helped it through various phases. Jag Ahluwahlia, a neonatologist at the Rosie Maternity Hospital, saw the value of what we were trying to prove and gave helpful advice throughout. German Berrios, chair of the Addenbrooke's Hospital Ethics Committee, helped us see the best way to carry out our study from the perspective of the mothers and children. Ian Goodyer and Joe Herbert, both professors in Cambridge with an interest in what hormones do to our brains, provided us with sound academic support. Melissa Hines in London, a leader in the field of hormones and behavior, provided helpful critiques of our work. Jenny Hannah, our wonderful secretary, gave us support in bringing the book to completion.

We are grateful to the Medical Research Council and the Gatsby Foundation for financial support of the research. In particular, the MRC funded Svetlana's doctoral thesis, from which much of the book is derived. Lastly, and most importantly, our thanks go to the mothers and children who have come back to our lab, year after year, to follow the plot with us.

1

Fetal Testosterone

Endocrine (hormonal) systems are involved in every aspect of pregnancy (including implantation, formation of the placenta, maternal adaptation, and embryonic and fetal development), in birth, and in adaptation to life outside the womb. Hormones have a range of functions involving reproduction, growth, and development, maintenance of the internal environment and the production, use, and storage of energy. Of greatest relevance to this book are the gonadal hormones, which are essential to the sexual differentiation of the fetus. This process includes sexual differentiation of the sex structures, as well as aspects of behavior and cognition (Hadley 2000; Wilson, Foster, Kronenberg, and Larsen 1998; Fuchs and Klopper 1983).

Gonadal Hormones

The gonadal hormones or sex steroids include androgens (e.g., testosterone, dihydrotestosterone), estrogens (e.g., estradiol, estrone, estriol), and progestins (e.g., progesterone). Progesterone is synthesized from cholesterol, and progesterone itself can subsequently be converted to testosterone. And testosterone is a precursor to estradiol and to dihydrotestosterone (Stryer 1995).

Figure 1.1 illustrates the chemical structures of several major gonadal hormones.

Four endocrine glands are capable of synthesizing sex hormones: the adrenals, the testes, the ovaries, and the placenta. The synthesis is the same in all these systems, but the end product of the synthesis depends on the target tissue—for example, the testes secrete testosterone, but the placenta uses it to make estradiol. The process by which testosterone is converted to estradiol is called *aromatization*.

Although estrogen is usually considered to be the female hormone and testosterone the male hormone, both hormones are present in both sexes. The sexes differ in the quantity of each hormone present and in the number of receptors for them (Hess et al. 1997). It is not only the availability of a hormone but also the sensitivity of the target tissue that determines the hormone's biological activity.

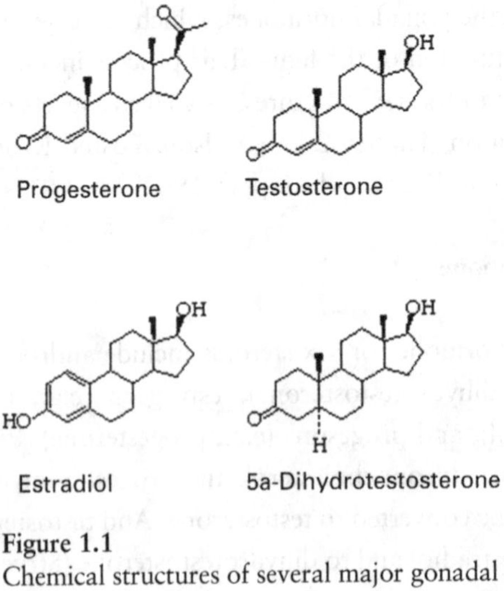

Progesterone   Testosterone

Estradiol   5a-Dihydrotestosterone

Figure 1.1
Chemical structures of several major gonadal hormones.

Androgens have a number of functions in humans. These include control of gonadotrophin production in the brain, initiation and maintenance of spermatogenesis, promotion of sexual maturity at puberty, control of sex drive, control of sexually dimorphic behavior patterns, and formation of the male phenotype during the sexual differentiation of the fetus. In addition to its involvement in sexual differentiation of the reproductive structures (known as its *androgenic effects*), testosterone is the major hormone responsible for sexual differentiation of such non-reproductive tissues as bone, muscle, kidney, and liver; these effects are called *anabolic* (Bardin and Catterall 1981).

Estrogens are involved in the development of female sexual secondary characteristics, development of the breasts and prevention of bone mineral loss. They have major differentiating effects on the reproductive tract, on the distribution of fat, and on certain bones (including the pelvis), but only minor effects on other organs (Bardin and Catterall 1981). Additionally, there is evidence that estrogens have a neuroprotective role during aging (Witelson 1991). Estrogens are important in the maintenance of pregnancy—for example, they are involved in the support of placental progesterone synthesis, in the increase and maintenance of maternal blood volume, and in the promotion of uterine growth (Repe and Albrecht 1990). There is also some evidence that estrogen has a role in implantation of the fertilized egg. Estrogens can have masculinizing as well as feminizing effects on development.

By week 3 or week 4 of gestation, the placenta is responsible for nearly all estrogen production in pregnancy. Some estrogen is produced by the fetal adrenal gland, which is active from around week 8. The fetal ovary produces little or no estrogen early in pregnancy. No ovarian estrogen synthesis can be detected until late in fetal life. Most of the estrogen is secreted into the maternal blood, but levels are also high in the fetus and in the amniotic fluid. The role of these high estrogen levels in the fetus is not yet clear. The most abundant estrogen is estriol, which is unique to pregnancy. It is mostly present in an inert form, so the fetus is protected from its potent effects. The mother has a high capacity for rendering estrogen inactive and so does not experience detrimental effects due to high estrogen production by the placenta.

Men normally produce about 100 times more testosterone than estradiol. Most of the estrogen is made from androgens, but the testes also secrete a small amount. Normally insignificant, this can become abnormal in certain medical conditions. Serum concentrations of estradiol are low in males, but they can be higher in semen than in the serum of females. Male reproductive tissues are known to express estrogen receptors, and there is evidence for a physiological role for estradiol in male reproductive function, related to the concentration of semen (Hess et al. 1997).

Progestins can be androgenic or anti-androgenic in their effects, depending on their chemical basis. Their effects are predictable, based on their chemical nature. For example, male-typical behaviors have been observed in females exposed prenatally to androgenic progestins (Collaer and Hines 1995). *Progesterone* is an anti-androgenic or progestational progestin. Progesterone has an essential role in pregnancy maintenance, affecting uterine musculature and inhibiting maternal immune responses to fetal cells.

Another important group of hormones is the *gonado-trophins*, including follicle-stimulating hormone (FSH) and luteinizing hormone (LH). Produced and released by the pituitary gland, these mediate the control of gonad function in both sexes. In males, FSH and LH are released in a constant, sustained manner and, in females, release is cyclic with a pre-ovulatory surge that leads to ovulation.

Alpha-fetoprotein (AFP), not a steroid hormone, merits discussion at the point because of its potential role in regulating the levels of steroid hormones. It is a globulin produced by the fetal liver and yolk sac during the first and second trimesters of pregnancy, from as early as week 4, and it is often measured during pregnancy (Gitlin, Pericelli, and Gitlin 1972).

Measurement of AFP in amniotic fluid is a reliable indicator of neural-tube defects between weeks 15 and 22 (Wathen, Campbell, Kitau, and Chard 1993). In such cases, maternal AFP levels tend to be high, as AFP leaks from the damaged fetus. In chromosomal disorders, low maternal serum levels could result from impaired fetal kidney function and impaired membrane or placental passage of AFP, rather than reduced fetal production (Van Lith et al. 1991).

AFP can be detected in the fetal brain after 12 weeks, with a peak value in week 20 (Ali, Balapure, Singh, Shukla, and Sahib 1981). Levels decline rapidly after week 24, after which AFP is absent. High levels are said to correspond to the period when critical hypothalamic differentiation is reported to occur in humans (Dörner 1978).

In placental mammals, the fetus is continually exposed to high levels of estrogens from the placenta and the mother. The protective mechanism from these high levels of hormones is well established in rodents. AFP binds to estrogen, but not to testosterone. However, AFP does not bind to estrogen in humans (MacLusky and Naftolin 1981). The mechanism by which the human fetus is protected from high levels of estrogens is not fully established.

The Placenta

The fetal hormone environment is dependent on a functioning placenta (Chara 1982) that regulates the exchange of molecules between the fetus and the mother. This means that the fetal environment is largely independent of maternal hormones, because the placenta is impermeable to most hormones. The placenta synthesizes estrogens, progesterone, polypeptide hormones, neuropeptides, and growth factors. The placenta has a very strong aromatizing enzyme system, and androgens tend to get converted to estrogen by it. This means that very little androgen is transmitted by the placenta.

Becoming Male or Staying Female: Sexual Differentiation of the Fetus

Gonadal hormones are responsible for differentiation of the male and female phenotypes in the developing human fetus (MacLusky and Naftolin 1981; Fuchs and Klopper 1983; Wilson et al. 1998; Kimura 1999), although direct genetic influences on sexual differentiation of the brain are increasingly recognized (Devries 2002, Arnold 1996). There are five major stages in normal sexual development.

The *genetic sex* is determined at the moment of conception by the presence of an X (female) or a Y (male) chromosome in the fertilizing sperm cell. The karyotype of the normal female is 46 XX; that of the normal male is 46 XY. Each is made up of 44 autosomes and 2 sex chromosomes. The male can be described as heterogametic, the female as homogametic. There are very few differences between the genes of males and females, except for the Y chromosome in the male (Bardin and Catterall 1981).

The genetic sex determines whether testes or ovaries develop (i.e. *gonadal sex*). Up until week 6, genetically male and genetically female fetuses are undifferentiated—that is, there is no difference between them with respect to their reproductive structures. During week 6, the Sry gene on the Y chromosome initiates testicular differentiation in the male; this is thought to be the major function of the Y chromosome. The Leydig cells of the testis are capable of synthesizing testosterone by the end of week 8. Further development of the Leydig cells means that testosterone secretion is high between weeks 10 and 20. Fetal synthesis of testosterone is probably controlled by hcG (human chorionic gonadotrophin) and LH from the fetal pituitary. In addition, males are exposed to fetal testosterone from the fetal adrenals.

In the female, differentiation of the ovaries begins around week 7. The fetal ovary may produce a small amount of estrogen (Smail, Reyes, Winter, and Faiman 1981). The female fetus is also exposed to low levels of androgens. A small proportion may come from the fetal adrenals, and some comes from the maternal adrenals, ovaries, and fat (Geschwind and Galaburda 1985b; Martin 1985).

The secretions of the gonads thus formed determine the *phenotypic sex*. If male sex hormones and the appropriate receptors are present, the male phenotype will develop; if sufficient male sex hormones or functioning receptors are not present (i.e., in females), the female phenotype will develop (Jost 1961; Jost 1972; Donahoe, Cate, and MacLaughlin 1987; George and Wilson 1992). The internal genitalia of both sexes are derived from the Wolffian (male) and Müllerian (female) ducts, which co-exist in the undifferentiated developing embryo. In the male, between weeks 8 and 14, the Wolffian ducts, stimulated by testosterone, develop into the male internal structures. The Müllerian ducts regress, thus preventing the formation of female internal structures. Regression of the Müllerian ducts is caused by anti-Müllerian hormone or Müllerian regression factor (secreted by the Sertoli cells of the testes). The formation of the male external genitalia is stimulated by dihydrotestosterone, which is formed from testosterone by 5-α-reductase. In the female, the absence of testosterone causes the Wolffian ducts to atrophy. The absence of anti-Müllerian hormone allows the Müllerian ducts to become the female internal structures. Similarly, the absence of male sex hormones allows female external genitalia to develop, rather than male structures.

Neuronal sex (which refers to male-type or female-type gonadotrophin secretion, sexual orientation, and gender role behavior) and *gender identity* (Dörner et al. 1987) are shaped to a large extent by prenatal factors.

In summary, masculinization requires the action of testicular hormones. The default mammalian sex is female, and in the absence of very high levels of male sex hormones female structures will develop. It has been assumed that no special hormonal environment is required for the formation of the female phenotype. That traditional model is now being replaced by a more complex one which recognizes that small amounts of ovarian hormones may be required for active feminization of the female brain (Beyer 1999). Still, many stages must be completed successfully if the male phenotype is to develop, and these stages rely to a large extent on the existence of the right hormonal environment. This implies that there are a number of stages at which the normal development of the male could be disrupted.

Not all animals have female as the default sex. In birds, for example, the default homogametic sex is male, and differentiation of the female depends on exposure to ovarian hormones. In mammals, fetuses are exposed to high levels of female hormones from the mother, so it is adaptive for the default sex to be female. In egg-laying species this does not apply, so having one sex as the default sex over the other does not necessarily confer the same advantages as in mammals (Hadley 2000). It is interesting to note that feminization of the brain in mammals by ovarian estrogen is thought to occur at a later period than masculinization (in female rats this may extend from the late neonatal to the pubertal period and perhaps even into adulthood) (Fitch 2002, p. 365). This would mean that ovarian-estrogen-mediated feminization takes place after the individual is free from the maternal-hormonal environment of the womb.

Organizational versus Activational Effects, and Sensitive Periods

Sex hormones have two different types of effect on tissue: organizational and activational (Goy and McEwen 1980). Organizational effects are permanent and happen early in development, usually during a sensitive period. Activational effects happen later in development and are superimposed on the early organizational effects. The later hormonal actions are necessary if the tissue or organ in question is to perform its function. For example, the tissues of the genetic male are organized prenatally for male adult reproductive behavior. However, the male will not display such behavior unless adequate sex hormones are produced at puberty. Although the dichotomy between organizational and activational effects is useful for understanding hormonal effects, it cannot always be rigidly applied (Arnold and Breedlove 1985). When studying the organizational effects of hormones on the developing fetus, it is important to remember that later activational effects may be essential to the function in question. For estrogen the distinction is particularly problematic, as estrogen appears to exert "organizational" effects for a very long period of time.

Both adult and fetal studies can be subject to the same criticism: the relationship between the time of measurement and the sensitive period for development is unknown. Sensitive (or critical) periods are hypothetical windows of time in which a tissue can be modified. Environmental disruptions during development can have devastating effects. A substance that causes damage curing a critical period may have no effect at all when development is complete. It is therefore adaptive to restrict development to specific, limited time periods. This means, for example, that circulating sex hormones necessary for adult sexual functioning do not cause unwanted alterations to tissues, even though the same hormones might have been essential to the development of those tissues. Different behaviors can have different sensitive periods for development. For example, androgen exposure early or late in gestation has differential effects on male typical juvenile behaviors in the female rhesus macaque (Goy, Bercovitch, and McBrair 1988).

Postnatal Hormone Surges

Neonatal

After the prenatal surge in testosterone production, there are two further testosterone surges in the human male. These occur neonatally and at puberty. Although the function of the neonatal surge is not fully understood in humans, it is likely to be related to the preparation of tissue for subsequent androgen mediated growth. In monkeys, disruption of the neonatal surge is known to lead to disrupted testicular function at puberty (Mann, Gould, and Collins 1989). As males may experience a testosterone surge at this time and females do not experience such a surge, the same amount of subsequent testosterone exposure will have very different effects on each sex (MacLusky and Naftolin 1981). Females experience a postnatal surge in estradiol production, which is thought to come from the ovaries (Bidlingmaier, Strom, Dorr, Eisenmenger, and Knorr 1987). Levels remain high for the first year of life, peaking around month 3 or 4. Median levels are equivalent to those in the second stage of puberty (Bidlingmaier, Versmold, and Knorr 1974). The postnatal surges in both sexes are stimulated by surges in gonadotrophin levels (Bidlingmaier et al. 1987).

Pubertal

Sexual differentiation is not complete until puberty, when secondary sexual characteristics develop and fertility is attained. The development of the gonads can be viewed as a continuum from the fetal stage to puberty, with reproduction as the ultimate goal.

Factors That Influence Testosterone Levels

The factors that influence testosterone levels, both prenatally and postnatally, include stress, alcohol use, smoking, and the spacing of births (Dorner et al. 1987).

Prenatal stress in male rats demasculinizes and feminizes adult sexual behavior (Ward 1977), and testosterone levels in newborn rats are reduced in stressed animals relative to non-stressed controls (Stahl, Gotz, Poppe, Amendt, and Dorner

1978). Human homosexual males report more stressors (such as bereavement) during their mother's pregnancy than controls (Dorner, Schenk, Schmiedel, and Ahrens 1983). In females, there is some evidence that prenatal stress is associated with male typical gender role and sexual behavior.

Testosterone and estradiol are also significantly decreased in alcohol users (Westney et al. 1991). Serum testosterone levels are positively correlated to smoking in mothers during pregnancy, and also in their adult daughters. Daughters' smoking during adolescence is influenced by mothers' smoking during pregnancy and by maternal testosterone levels during pregnancy. In addition, maternal testosterone during pregnancy influences daughters' testosterone level, so this could be one mechanism whereby testosterone levels are transmitted from one generation to the next (Kandel and Udry 1999).

Hormone levels during a pregnancy are also influenced by how recently the mother has had a child. First-borns of both sexes have higher estrogen and progesterone levels, and male first-borns have higher testosterone than later-borns, when these are measured in umbilical-cord blood. This is not due to maternal age, length of labor, or birth weight. Close spacing of childbirths (i.e., less than 4 years) results in lower-than-normal hormone levels. The reduction in hormone levels is greater when the fetuses are male. After 4 years, levels are at first-born levels or higher (Maccoby, Doering, Jacklin, and Kraemer 1979).

2

Why Study Fetal Testosterone?

Studying fetal testosterone in humans has the potential to inform several areas of research.

Sex Differences in Cognition and Behavior

A large number of studies have reported cognitive and behavioral differences between men and women, on average. The general picture is that as a group men are typically stronger at non-verbal spatial tasks and that as a group women are stronger at verbal and social tasks. Kimura (1999) summarizes some of the major findings from the sex differences literature concerning motor skills, spatial and mathematical ability and verbal skills. In general, findings indicate that on average men are superior at targeting and women at fine motor skills. Men tend to navigate using spatial cues; women rely more on landmarks and have a superior memory for object location. The most reliable sex difference on spatial tasks is found in studies of mental rotation (Linn and Petersen 1985). In mathematics, men tend to be stronger at problem solving and reasoning, women stronger at computation (Geary 1996). With regard to verbal abilities, women tend to have better verbal memory, spelling ability, and verbal fluency, although their vocabularies are not larger than those of men. Developmentally however, a number of studies have reported greater vocabularies and faster rates of language acquisition in girls (Fenson et al. 1994; Huttenlocher, Haight, Bryk, Seltzer, and Lyons 1991; Hyde and Linn 1988; Reynell and Huntley 1985). Sex differences in emotion perception have been revealed on tasks where children are required to attribute subtle mental states to a person—for example, when interpreting the eye region of the face (Baron-Cohen, Jolliffe, Mortimore, and Robertson 1997).

In the field of cerebral lateralization, some studies support the idea that females are less lateralized for some cognitive function than males. On the basis of a review of a small number of dichotic listening studies, McGlone (1980) concluded that females were more symmetric than males on tests of dichotic listening. Hiscock, Inch, Jacek, Hiscock-Kalil, and Kalil (1993) found that 9 of 11 relevant studies supported the same conclusion. Such findings support the idea that women are less lateralized for language than men. If language is represented in both hemispheres in women, this might account for female superiority on some verbal tasks (Levy 1976).

Crucian and Berenbaum (1998) tested if the right hemisphere was organized for emotion perception in women and for spatial ability in men. The expected sex differences were observed on tests of emotional and spatial processing, but there was no inverse correlation between performance on the two types of task. This result suggests that one of the two skills does not develop at the expense of the other. In contrast, Jarrold (1998, p. 384) found a significant negative correlation between speed on the embedded figures task (a spatial test on which men usually outperform women) and the ability to identify emotional expressions (as measured by Baron-Cohen's "eyes task" (Baron-Cohen et al. 2001), which shows a female superiority) in a group of 60 undergraduates (30 male, 30 female). This suggests that some sex differences may be related reciprocally.

Witelson (1976) examined the development of lateralization for spatial ability in 200 girls and boys between the ages of 6 and 13 years. Children were required to palpate two meaningless objects (that could not readily be labeled) simultaneously and out of sight. They then had to choose the two objects from a visual array. Boys were better with their left hand (right hemisphere) than their right hand. Girls showed no difference between their hands, and there was no sex difference in overall accuracy. By the age of 6 years, boys were showing right hemisphere superiority on a spatial task. Girls were showing bilateral representation until at least adolescence. This could be indicative of greater plasticity in females for longer, which some have surmised might protect them against developmental disorders caused by early brain damage (ibid.).

Sex Differences in the Brain

There is a great deal of evidence for sexual dimorphism in the central nervous system, at the cellular level, in synaptic or dendritic organization, and in the gross volume of defined cell groups, and most of these features are thought to depend on early sex hormones (MacLusky and Naftolin 1981; Collaer and Hines 1995; Witelson 1991). Male sex hormones play a major role in the formation of sexually dimorphic structures in the rat brain, including the sexually dimorphic nucleus of the preoptic area or SDN-POA (a part of the hypothalamus) and the hippocampus. In humans, sex differences have been reported in the hypothalamus, the amygdala, and the cortex.

The hypothalamus is one of the most widely recognized areas of the brain to show a sex difference (Kimura 1999). It is important for general life functions, including eating, sleeping, and reproduction. A human equivalent of the rat SDN-POA was described by Swaab and Fliers (1985). Swaab and Hofman (1988) reported evidence from a human study that the sex difference in this region was apparent only after 2–4 years of age. Allen, Hines, Shryne, and Gorski (1989) reported that the area named as the SDN-POA by Swaab and Fliers should be referred to as "INAH-1"—i.e., the interstitial nucleus of the anterior hypothalamus, labeled 1 to distinguish it from the other INAHs. INAH-2 and INAH-3 were said to be bigger in males than in females, but INAH-1 (the SDN-POA equivalent) was not. LeVay (1991) reported a sex difference in INAH-3, but not in INAH-1 or INAH-2. However, INAH-3 was found to be larger in heterosexual men than in homosexual men.

Sexual dimorphism is also observed in the amygdala. One study of 15 human males and 15 human females between the ages of 7 and 11 found that the amygdala was smaller in the females (Caviness, Kennedy, Richelme, Rademacher, and Filipek 1996). In contrast, Murphy and Greer (1986) found no evidence for a sex difference. In rats, testosterone implants in the amygdala from day 1 of life resulted in a more masculine pattern of play fighting (Meaney and McEwen 1986). This indicated that a sex difference in the amygdala might mediate sex differences in play fighting.

Another region of the brain that has been well documented to show sexual dimorphism is the cortex. Regions of interest are the sylvian fissure and planum temporale (Aboitiz et al.

1992). The planum temporale is the brain region lying posterior to the primary auditory cortex. In about two-thirds of adults it is larger on the left; in the remaining third, it is either symmetrical or larger on the right. Deviations from the more standard pattern occur more commonly in women than men (Wada, Clarke, and Hamm 1975). There is reportedly an anatomical asymmetry in the sylvian fissure at 16 weeks, before any sex receptors are present in the cortex (LeMay and Culebras 1972).

Other brain features reported to show sexual dimorphism include the thickness of the cortex (Collaer and Hines 1995), the corpus callosum, brain weight at birth (Pakkenberg and Gundersen 1997; Pakkenberg and Voigt 1964), and the size of the prefrontal and the tempero-parietal cortex (Witelson 1991). The massa intermedia, which connects the right and left thalamus, is absent more often in males than in females (Lansdell and Davie 1972). Additionally, the frontal and occipital protuberances (i.e., the amount that one hemisphere protrudes beyond the other at the frontal and occipital poles) are larger in males (Bear, Schiff, Saver, Greenberg, and Freeman 1986).

If prenatal hormones are to act on the developing brain, the relevant brain regions must have available receptors. An understanding of where these receptors exist (and when in development) can help clarify the action of prenatal hormones on the brain. One study of male and female rat brains revealed that the most consistent sex differences in androgen receptors were in the amygdala and the hypothalamus (Meaney, Aitken, Jensen, McGinnis, and McEwen 1985). A study of rhesus monkeys found evidence for androgen binding sites identical to those in the genital tract, in the arcuate lateral septal, premammillary and intercalated mammillary nuclei. Estrogen binding sites were found in medial preoptic nuclei, in ventromedial hypothalamic nuclei, and in accessory basal amygdaloid nuclei (Michael, Rees, and Bonsall 1989). A small postmortem study of pre- and post-menopausal female brains found the highest concentration of testosterone and estradiol in the hypothalamus (Bixo, Backstrom, Winblad, and Andersson 1995); this may reflect the availability of receptors in those regions. Abramovich (1974) carried out a small study of the uptake of labeled testosterone by the fetal hypothalamus at 12–18 weeks and compared it to the cerebellum. Greater uptake was observed by hypothalamus. Abramovich pointed out that testosterone levels in the plasma of the male fetus remain high well after the differentiation of the genitalia, which supported the idea that high levels of pre-natal sex hormones are important for differentiation of the brain.

Hormonal Actions on the Brain

There is a great deal of evidence, especially from animal studies, that sex hormones act directly on the brain. In rodents, andro-gens seem to have many but not all of their effects on the brain by first being aromatized to estradiol (MacLusky 1981; Hadley 2000). For mammals other than rodents, the extent to which masculization is mediated by estrogens rather than androgens is unclear. Among non-human primates there is little evidence for an effect of estrogen on rough-and-tumble play or reproductive behaviors. Instead, it is testosterone or its metabolite dihy-drotestosterone (DHT) acting on androgen receptors that alters the expression of these behaviors (Breedlove 1994, p. 170; Goy et al. 1998). In addition, some humans are born without func-tioning androgen receptors, a condition known as androgen insensitivity (AI). Even if they are genetic males and secrete testosterone, they develop as phenotypic females. This further suggests that testosterone or dihydrotestosterone acting on the androgen receptor is the primary method of masculinization in primates, including humans. Nevertheless, it is important to keep in mind both the potential masculinizing and the potential feminizing effects of estradiol on development.

3

Cerebral Lateralization and Animal Studies

Most individuals exhibit the standard dominance pattern for cerebral lateralization—that is, specialization of the left hemisphere for language and handedness (i.e., right-handedness) and specialization of the right hemisphere for the processing of nonverbal information. In a study of children and adults that examined manual preference for a range of tasks, Annett (1967, 1998) estimated that approximately 3–4 percent of the population were strongly left-handed, 25–33 percent showed mixed handedness, and 60–70 percent were strongly right-handed. Studies of individuals with unilateral brain lesions resulting in aphasia have been carried out to estimate the proportion of people with left-hemisphere and right-hemisphere specialization for language. Grimshaw, Bryden, and Finegan (1995a) cite estimates that 61 percent of left-handers have left-hemisphere specialization for language, 20 percent have language served by both hemispheres, and 19 percent have right-hemisphere language. According to Segalowitz and Bryden (1983), 95 percent of right-handers show left-hemisphere specialization for language. Annett (1985) examined the results of four studies of aphasic patients and found that the average proportion of right-hemisphere lesions (implying right-hemisphere language) was just over 9 percent. Knecht et al. (2000) examined language lateralization in 188 healthy right-handed individuals by measuring blood flow in each hemisphere during a word-generation task. They observed that the natural distribution of language lateralization occurred along a bimodal continuum, that there was no sex difference in lateralization, and that right-hemisphere dominance for language was present in 7.5 percent of the children. Techniques such as presentation of visual material to one visual field only (assuming processing by the contralateral hemisphere) have demonstrated a right-hemisphere advantage for nonverbal material (McGlone 1980).

Individuals vary in the degree to which they show hemispheric specialization for particular skills, and it is generally accepted that individual differences in one dimension (e.g., handedness) may be independent of individual differences in another dimension (e.g., spatial skills) (Schafer and Plunkett 1998). Individual differences in cerebral lateralization are said to result in observable differences between individuals—for example, some individuals are more strongly left-handed than others.

It is also hypothesized that sex differences in cerebral lateralization account for some observable sex differences in behavior and cognition (Hines and Shipley 1984)—for example, a higher incidence of left-handedness in males than in females (Annett 1985). One study of 80 women assessed handedness and sex-typed personality characteristics (Nicholls and Forbes 1996). A "physiological" questionnaire was employed to examine bra size, age of menarche (first menstrual period), and regularity of menstruation. Left-handed women tended to have more masculine personality characteristics than right-handers, but right-handers and left-handers did not differ on the physiological measures apart from a non-significant pattern of less regular menses in the left-handers. This study gives some indication that left-handedness (which is more common in males) can be linked with masculinization and defeminization in females.

Therefore, an understanding of the processes that underlie individual differences in cerebral lateralization should help us to understand sex differences in cerebral lateralization, and ultimately sex differences in behavior and cognition. One possible agent leading to individual differences in cerebral lateralization is fetal testosterone (FT). Levels of FT differ between the sexes and also between individuals within each sex and so could be related to between-sex and within-sex differences, particularly on sexually dimorphic behaviors.

Theories of Cerebral Lateralization

The Callosal Hypothesis
The corpus callosum connects the two hemispheres. Its main functional role may be the transfer of already encoded information between homologous cortical areas (Kertesz, Polk, Howell, and Black 1987). The Callosal Hypothesis states that cerebral lateralization results from pruning of callosal cells during fetal and neonatal development, and that this process is mediated at least in part by testosterone (Witelson and Nowakowski 1991). This means that increased FT activity will result in a smaller corpus callosum, decreased connectivity between the hemispheres (especially in the tempero-parietal region), and greater lateralization of cognitive functions.

Some supporting evidence comes from post-mortem studies which showed that consistently right-handed men had smaller corpus callosa than inconsistent right-handers, thus suggesting that variation in lateralization may indeed be related to callosal size. Increased left-handedness was said to arise from greater connectivity between the two hemispheres. This effect was not observed in women, and it was thought that different mechanisms might apply to each sex (Witelson and Goldsmith 1991; Witelson 1985). This work has been criticized for its low subject numbers and lack of true left-handers in the sample (Kertesz et al. 1987).

Sexual dimorphism has been reported in studies of the corpus callosum. One post-mortem study of 9 males and 5 females found that the posterior part of the corpus callosum (the splenium) was larger in females than in males (De Lacoste-Utamsing and Holloway 1982). This was confirmed by Holloway, Anderson, Defendini, and Harper (1993). Additionally, the average callosal area was found to be greater in females than males (De Lacoste-Utamsing and Holloway 1982), and this was partially supported by Holloway et al. (1993). If a greater callosal area means a greater number of callosal fibers (an assumption for which there is some support—see Aboitiz, Scheibel, and Zaidel 1992), the findings suggest that females may have greater connectivity between the two hemispheres than males. This would be consistent with the idea that females are less lateralized for cognitive functions than males (McGlone 1980). This is because increased connectivity means that information can be shared more easily between the hemispheres, rather than being restricted to just one.

Further support for the role of callosal axon loss in the etiology of cerebral lateralization comes from studies of premature babies. Children whose birth weights were less than 1,000 grams were found to be more left-handed at the age of 4 years (corrected for prematurity) than those whose birth weights were greater than 1,000 grams. Those babies with the lower birth weights were born very early (weeks 26–29), which may have resulted in interference with normal axonal pruning, leading to a larger corpus callosum (as in the non-right-handed men in the Witelson studies) and increased left-handedness. The sexes of the children were not noted (O'Callaghan et al. 1987).

A study in which magnetic-resonance imaging was used to examine the corpus callosa of 104 children challenges the Callosal Hypothesis. The study failed to find a convincing sex difference or a significant difference between handedness groups (Kertesz et al. 1987). The same study measured cerebral dominance on a dichotic listening task and a visual half-field task, in which words were presented to one visual field only. There was no relationship between callosal size and lateralization of auditory or visual language processing. An additional challenge comes from an alternative hypothesis that a larger corpus callosum means that the two hemispheres will inhibit each other and therefore result in greater lateralization of function (Aboitiz et al. 1992; Zaidel, Clarke, and Suyenobu 1990).

A major implication of the Callosal Hypothesis is that reduced FT (associated with decreased axonal pruning) is associated with increased left-handedness and less functional asymmetry (i.e., reduced lateralization). Some support for this prediction comes from evidence outlined by Witelson (1991) that Kleinfelter's Syndrome is associated with lower testosterone levels in early development, but also with increased left-handedness. This prediction is opposite to that of Norman Geschwind, who associated increased FT levels with increased left-handedness.

There are no human data currently available on the relationship between prenatal testosterone levels and callosal size.

Data of this sort are needed in order for the Callosal Hypothesis to be tested properly. One study of 68 young adult right-handed males found a positive correlation between salivary testosterone levels and the cross-sectional area of the posterior body of the corpus callosum (Moffat, Hampson, Wickett, Vernon, and Lee 1997). The Callosal Hypothesis would presumably predict an inverse correlation between testosterone and callosal size. However, the Moffat study looked at salivary testosterone levels, rather than prenatal levels, so the results are inconclusive.

Some studies have looked at the effect of sex hormones on the corpus callosum in rats. In the rat, it is the male that has a larger corpus callosum (Fitch, Cowell, Schrott, and Denenberg 1991). Neonatal testosterone injections have been found to masculinize the corpus callosum of the female, while neonatal castration does not appear to affect the male (Nunez and Juraska 1998). Prenatal testosterone levels appear to be the critical factor in the male (Mack, McGivern, Hyde, and Denenberg 1996). The size of the splenium is increased in females from litters with a high male-to-female ratio (Nunez and Juraska 1998), suggesting an effect of exposure to higher levels of male sex hormones in utero. Additionally, there is evidence that ovarian hormones actively feminize the corpus callosum in the female rat, and that masculinization and feminization of the corpus callosum are two distinct processes, with different sensitive periods (Fitch et al. 1991).

The Geschwind Hypothesis
The Geschwind Hypothesis addresses the biological mechanisms of lateralization (Geschwind and Behan 1982; Geschwind and Galaburda 1985a,b,c). This hypothesis was formulated to

account for six observations: increased left-handedness in males relative to females, the elevated rate in males relative to females of the developmental disorders of language and speech, female superiority at verbal tasks and male superiority at spatial tasks, superior right-hemisphere functions in left-handers and individuals with developmental disorders, the elevated rate of non-right-handedness in developmental disorders, and the elevated rate of immune disorders in non-right-handers.

Other experimental findings that inspired Geschwind's work (summarized in Geschwind and Galaburda 1985a) were concerned with anatomic and chemical asymmetries in the brain (both prenatally and postnatally), with cell death in the developing brain, with reorganization of the brain after intra-uterine lesions, with hormonal influences on brain structures, and with genetic studies of handedness and the evolution of asymmetry as evidenced by fossil skulls. An additional area of interest was patterns of maturation in the brain. The male brain was said to mature later than the female brain, and the left hemisphere later than the right.

In summary, the Geschwind Hypothesis suggests that testosterone acts during a critical period of brain development and slows the growth of certain areas of the left hemisphere, especially the temporal speech region. This growth retardation may be sufficient to shift some left-hemisphere functions (e.g., language and handedness) to the right hemisphere. Additionally, the growth of adjacent areas on the left may be enhanced. A continuum of laterality is proposed in which language and handedness are initially established on the left, perhaps genetically. This suggests that the fundamental pattern of the brain involves a strong asymmetry, and Geschwind supported the idea that asymmetry is present in the ovum (Corballis and

Morgan 1978). Increased exposure to FT then shifts lateralization increasingly to the right. FT is said to influence the developing immune system, accounting for the associations between immune functioning and laterality. Geschwind acknowledged that other prenatal and postnatal factors (e.g., length of gestation or timing of puberty) could have a role in cerebral lateralization, but Geschwind's emphasis was on the intra-uterine environment. If there is indeed asymmetry in the ovum, this shows that there must be a non-hormonal component to the final patterns of asymmetry achieved.

Males obviously are exposed to more testosterone prenatally than females. Serum measurements of testosterone from week 12 to week 18 show males with an average of 249 ng/100 ml (±93) and females with an average 29 ng/100 ml (±19) (Abramovich 1973, p. 261). This means that there will be more left-sided growth retardation in males and a greater shift to the right hemisphere. This would account for findings of increased left-handedness in males relative to females. Critical to the hypothesis is the fact that females are also exposed to small amounts of testosterone. If not, the hypothesis could not account for variability between females. Geschwind pointed out that the effects of testosterone depend on the availability of free unbound hormone and on the sensitivity of target tissues. (If a tissue has no receptors, it will not react even to large doses of hormone.)

When the Geschwind Hypothesis was first published, it generated a great deal of interest, largely because it touched on many areas of biology and medicine. Researchers attempted to test the predictions of the theory by looking at associations between, for example, handedness and immune disorders, or handedness and developmental disorders. Although many early citations of the theory were uncritical (McManus and Bryden 1991), the theory is generally not accepted now, at least not in its entirety. Small parts of it have been readily refuted as studies have failed to support its predictions (Bryden, McManus, and Bulman 1994). One study, for example, concluded that left-handedness was not directly related to either learning disorders or immune disorders and that concepts such as "learning disorders" and "immune disorders" needed to be more clearly defined (Obrzut 1994). Other concepts, including "anomalous dominance," were also found to be poorly defined (McManus and Bryden 1991). Additionally, the Geschwind Hypothesis does not make any mention of activational effects of hormones. The Geschwind Hypothesis has drawn attention to the importance of the prenatal environment to brain development, and ultimately psychological development.

The Advantages of a Lateralized Brain

Cerebral lateralization allows an individual to possess more skills than that individual would have if a given skill had to be replicated in both hemispheres. Modification of lateralization by prenatal factors allows for greater diversity than if lateralization were to be predetermined purely genetically. This maximization of diversity is adaptive for survival (Geschwind and Galaburda 1985a).

The right hemisphere matures before the left (ibid.), which means that it will be less subject to disrupting influences during development. This is important, as the right hemisphere has a special role in the processes essential to survival, such as attention and analysis of external space and emotion (ibid.).

Animal Studies

A large number of animal studies have examined the effect of prenatal hormones on postnatal outcome. They lend a great deal of support to the view that exposure to masculine prenatal hormones organizes the brain for masculine postnatal behavior. There is an argument that the study of animal models does not provide useful insights into human pregnancy. However, the animal models clearly are useful for highlighting potential areas of interest and for the guidance of predictions. In addition, Kimura (1999) points out that the discovery of sex differences in animal models is highly informative, as male and female lab animals are generally not treated differently by the researchers. However, social influences are not entirely lacking in animal models. For example, mother rats lick the anogenital regions of their male pups more than their female pups, a behavior that stimulates evacuation reflexes of the bladder and the colon. Variations in maternal care have long-term effects on offspring's behavior and the anatomy of the nervous system.

The areas investigated by animal studies include the effect of hormones on neuroanatomy and on non-reproductive and reproductive behavior. In the male rat, for example, the right cortex is observed to be thicker on the right than on the left, and the opposite is true in the female. The female pattern can be produced in males if they are castrated at birth (Diamond 1984). The sexually dimorphic nucleus of the preoptic area (SDN-POA) of the hypothalamus is known to be important for sexual behavior and is larger in male rats than in females. Early androgen injections in the female can masculinize the SDN-POA (Arnold and Gorski 1984).

In the field of non-reproductive behavior, testosterone injections 4 days after birth made male gerbils show a feminized pattern of forepaw use. In females, the same behavior was either masculinized or feminized, depending on the dosage (Clark, Robertson, and Galef 1996). One study found that the spatial maze navigation of male rats could be feminized by neonatal castration and that of female rats could be masculinized by early estradiol injections (Williams, Barnett, and Meck 1990). Female rats tend to use landmark cues for navigation, whereas males tend to use spatial cues. A further study of non-reproductive behavior found that the perinatal testosterone surge in male rhesus monkeys temporarily slowed the maturation of the neural system underlying performance on a visual task (Bachevalier, Hagger, and Bercu 1989).

One well-known area of investigation concerning courtship behavior is singing in birds. Male zebra finches sing much more than females, and their neural "song centers" are 5–6 times larger than those of females (Nottebohm and Arnold 1976). Early estrogen treatment of females was found to masculinize the song centers, and females would sing in adulthood, but only if given an activational dose of androgens (Gurney and Konishi 1980). The canary brain, in contrast, remains "plastic" into adulthood, and androgen treatment in the adult female will produce some changes in the song nuclei (Goldman and Nottebohm 1983). Disruption of hormones in the male has not been found to prevent the male songbird system from forming. This indicates that there might be a genetic non-hormonal mechanism in place to achieve the final adult pattern (Arnold 1997). It is worth considering the existence of such mechanisms in other species, and for other behaviors.

The more direct effects of hormones on mating behavior have also been studied in birds. A study of female zebra finches found that early estradiol injections and subsequent testosterone implants could lead to a masculinized pattern of mate choice (i.e., preference for a female mate), but only if the birds lived in a single-sex setting during their early life. This suggested that sexual partner preference (an important sexually dimorphic component of mate choice) was organized by sex steroids in a way that was mediated by the environment (Mansukhani, Adkins-Regan, and Yang 1996). In a more recent study, Adkins-Regan (1999) found that sexual preference was still masculinized, even if the later testosterone treatment was not administered.

Sexual behavior has also been studied in rodents. For example, early testosterone injections have been found to masculinize sexual behavior in rats (Harris and Levine 1962). Matuszczyk and Larsson (1995) concluded that prenatal estrogen is involved in the development of mechanisms involved in the display of male-typical behaviors in adulthood, in the suppression of female-typical behavior, and in the stimulation of neural mechanisms influencing sexual preference behavior in the adult. Prenatal treatment with anti-estrogen abolished the capacity of the male adult to ejaculate and enhanced the potential to exhibit female type sexual behavior. That is, female-oriented behavior was reduced in a two-choice stimulus situation between an estrous female and active male.

The evidence discussed in this chapter provides clear support for the idea that fetal testosterone affects cerebral lateralization, subsequent brain development, and subsequent behavior.

4

Disorders of Sexual Development

As we described earlier, there are three major stages in normal sexual differentiation. If one of these stages is disrupted, the result is disordered sexual differentiation (Hadley 2000; Collaer and Hines 1995; Grimshaw et al. 1995a; Grumbach and Conte 1992).

The disorders can be divided into two broad categories: disorders of sex determination and disorders of sex differentiation. Disorders of sex determination are most often caused by sex chromosome abnormalities or gene abnormalities affecting gonadogenesis, and disorders of sex differentiation are often characterized by an abnormal hormonal environment. The abnormality can be due to genetic or environmental factors. This second group of conditions is the most relevant to the study of prenatal hormones, as cognitive and behavioral studies of affected individuals can provide insight into the role of hormones in development.

One condition associated with an anomalous hormonal environment is congenital adrenal hyperplasia (CAH). A genetic defect results in the production of high levels of androgens beginning in the third month of gestation. Cases normally are identified at birth; treatment is then begun. Therefore,

androgen production is continuously high only during the prenatal period. Females with CAH are typically born with masculinized external genitalia, which can be surgically corrected
in infancy, and CAH is said to be the most common cause of
ambiguous genitalia at birth (Hughes 1998). The outward
signs in males are less obvious. Patients are treated with corti-
sol-replacement therapy (as cortisol deficiency is causal), and
with salt-retaining measures in the salt-wasting form of the disorder. Successful treatment means that excessive androgenization is limited to the prenatal and early postnatal periods.

Collaer and Hines (1995) cite a study (New and Levine
1984) that estimates CAH to affect between 1/5,000 and
1/15,000 of births. Although CAH can affect both males and
females, the most interesting psychological findings have come
from studies of females, who are usually compared to unaffected female relatives. This is probably because boys with
CAH experience androgenization in the high but normal range.
A number of these findings are outlined by Grimshaw et al.
(1995a) and by Collaer and Hines (1995). These findings
include increased bisexual and homosexual fantasies and experience (Dittman, Kappes, and Kappes 1992), a less strong
female identity (Zucker et al. 1996), masculinization of certain
attitudes (Dittman et al. 1990), increased left-handedness (Nass
et al. 1987), and increased visuo-spatial skills (Hampson,
Rovet, and Altmann 1994). Increased levels of language disabilities have been documented in CAH patients and their families (Plante, Boliek, Binkiewicz, and Erly 1996). Plante et al.
(ibid.) have also reported an increased rate of atypical brain
symmetry, as measured by magnetic-resonance imaging.

Other studies have failed to support the idea of masculinization in CAH. Helleday, Siwers, Ritzen, and Hugdahl (1994)

reported that females with CAH did not differ from controls on hand preference or dichotic listening asymmetry, Baker and Ehrhard (1974) reported no difference on tests of visuo-spatial ability; they also noted deficits in quantitative ability that would not be predicted by a simple theory of testosterone-produced masculinization. In addition, females with CAH were found not to differ from their unaffected sisters in assertiveness, dominance, acceptance in peer groups, or energy expenditure (Dittman et al. 1990).

Negative findings do not mean that elevated androgen exposure in CAH does not lead to a more masculine pattern of lateralization. It is not necessary for all measurable aspects of behavior and cognition to be masculinized in order for the theory to be correct. Additionally, one task that aims to measure a certain skill might reveal masculinization, whereas another might not. It is important for interpretation of studies to know exactly what we mean by, for example, "visuo-spatial skills."

Another disorder of sexual differentiation is idiopathic hypogonadotrophic hypogonadism (IHH), which affects genetically normal males. Gonadal steroid production is reduced by inadequate stimulation of the testes, caused either by reduced pituitary gonadotrophin levels or by their hypothalamic releasing factor. IHH can be congenital or can develop later in life. At birth external genitalia are normal, probably due to stimulation of the testes by maternal gonadotrophins. One study compared 19 men with IHH, 19 normal controls, and 5 men who had developed the condition later in life. The IHH children were found to show impaired performance on spatial tasks relative to the other two groups, and performance was correlated to testicular volume, which is assumed to be inversely related to the severity of the condition. The spatial tasks used were the Block Design Test, the Embedded Figures Test, and the Spatial Relations Subtest from the Differential Aptitude Tests. Androgen-replacement therapy in six of the IHH children did not improve their performance, which implied that prenatal conditions were critical. These late-onset cases would have been exposed to normal prenatal testosterone levels (Hier and Crowley 1982).

Another example of disordered sexual differentiation is anorchia, in which testes are present early in neonatal life but later disappear due to trauma or vascular damage. Although differentiation of the male genitalia can be normal (as it occurs while the testes are still present), subsequent surges in testosterone production are absent. Androgen insensitivity (AI) occurs when there is a partial or complete deficit of androgen receptors. At birth, males with this condition are phenotypically normal females; in older children, there is evidence for a feminized pattern of performance on visuo-spatial tasks. It is interesting that some children with AI show left-handedness. This supports the idea that there is some other route to left-handedness besides FT action (Imperato-McGinley, Pichardo, Gautier, Voyer, and Bryden 1991). However, it is also possible that FT exerts some effects in these individuals by first being converted to estradiol, for which receptors are believed to be intact in AI (Hampson and Moffat 1994). Individuals with Turner's Syndrome and Kleinfelter's Syndrome have also been studied. Both of these conditions are associated with abnormal sex chromosomes and extensive clinical problems, so their study is less relevant to the relationship between prenatal hormones and normal psychological development than the study of some other individuals.

The hormonal environment of the fetus can be disrupted by external factors, such as ingestion of synthetic hormones by the mother. One such synthetic hormone is diethylstilbestrol (DES), which was administered to women to assist with pregnancy maintenance from the 1940s to the 1970s. In one study by Hines and Shipley, 25 females who had been exposed to DES in utero were compared to their unaffected sisters. Children had to have been exposed to DES for at least 5 months of pregnancy, including the entire second trimester, in order to increase the likelihood that exposure occurred during the critical period for lateralization. Additionally, children had to be at least 14 years of age and menstruating, as sex differences have been said to be more reliably observed after puberty (Maccoby and Jacklin 1974). Verbal and visuo-spatial ability were assessed using tests that are known to yield sex differences; however, no differences were observed between the DES females and their sisters. Some aspects of a dichotic listening task, carried out with 13 of the sib pairs, yielded a more masculine pattern of results in the DES children than in the controls. That is, the left-ear and right-ear performances of the DES children were negatively correlated and their right-ear scores exceeded their left-ear scores. The effect of sex had been established in a pilot study in which normal males performed more like the DES children and normal females performed more like the unaffected sisters. The pilot males had a greater laterality index (i.e., degree of cerebral lateralization) than the pilot females, but there was no difference between the DES group and the control sisters on this measure (Hines and Shipley 1984). In another study, involving 10 DES exposed males and their unaffected brothers, DES exposure was found to be associated with a feminized pattern of reduced hemispheric laterality and with lowered spatial ability (Reinisch and Sanders 1992).

There are several ways in which sexual differentiation can go wrong. Although disordered sexual differentiation may not always be outwardly obvious at birth, it can have later implications for fertility and can affect developmental outcome. Studies of individuals with these conditions demonstrate that the prenatal hormone environment can influence behavior and cognition. However, it may not be useful to generalize the results to the non-clinical population. In part, this is because studies are necessarily carried out with small samples—for example, Hier and Crowley (1982) studied 19 patients and 24 controls, Dittman et al. (1990) 35 patients and 16 controls, and Zucker et al. (1996) 31 patients and 15 controls. A further reason is that it is impossible to differentiate between the effects of the hormonal environment and those of any gene abnormalities associated with the disorder. Also, because the hormone levels involved are abnormal, they might lead to abnormal patterns of development, which do not relate well to normal development. Additionally, a procedure such as corrective surgery for ambiguous genitalia may have a great impact on patients and their families, influencing the socialization of the patient. Finally, the above studies are not truly experimental, in that children could obviously not be randomly assigned to treatment groups (Hines and Shipley 1984).

Sex Bias in Disorders

Some developmental disorders and some behaviors occur more commonly in males than in females. These include the autism spectrum conditions (Skuse 2000; Wing 1981), language delay, attention deficit with hyperactivity disorder (ADHD), criminality, and antisocial behavior (Lord and Schopler 1987). Autism research, in particular, has yielded findings that are consistent with the idea that male sex hormones may be implicated in its etiology.

Testosterone and Autism: Any Links?

The first piece of evidence that links autism to "maleness" is the striking ratio of males to females among individuals with the condition. The sex ratio of males to females reported in the literature ranges from approximately 2:1 to 4:1 (Lord and Schopler 1987; Wing 1981), and approximately 9 times as many males as females are diagnosed with Asperger's Syndrome (which can be viewed as a milder form of autism). The exact ratio depends somewhat on the inclusion criteria adopted—such as excluding severely retarded individuals or using a broad definition of autism. A second link to maleness comes from cognitive studies of autism. Experimental findings have led to the suggestion that autism is an extreme form of the male brain (Baron-Cohen 2000; Baron-Cohen and Hammer 1997). These findings include reports that individuals with autism are superior to controls on tasks that normally give rise to male superiority (e.g., the Embedded Figures Task—see Jolliffe and Baron-Cohen 1997 and Shah and Frith 1983) and impaired on tasks that normally give rise to female superiority (e.g., the Reading the Mind in the Eyes Task—see Baron-Cohen, Jolliffe, Mortimore, and Robertson 1997). One candidate mechanism for this association of autism and being male is the action of prenatal male sex hormones. This idea that autism might be linked to high levels of prenatal testosterone was also a part of the Geschwind Hypothesis. Fetal testosterone was hypothesized to cause hemispheric abnormalities underlying the cognitive characteristics of autism.

Other research, which has looked more directly at hormones in autism, has further highlighted a possible link between autism and testosterone. Findings include observations of hypermasculinization (Hermle and Oepen 1987) and precocious puberty (Tordjman and Ferrari 1992) in clinical patients with autism. Additionally, a link between aggression in autism and abnormally high androgen levels has been observed (Tordjman, Ferrari, Sulmont, Duyme, and Roubertoux 1997) as well as macro-orchidism and sex hormone abnormalities in Fragile X (which is associated with autistic features) (Bregman, Dykens, Watson, Ort, and Leckman 1987).

One study of 39 pre-pubertal and post-pubertal males with autism reported that their plasma testosterone levels did not differ significantly from those of 12 mentally handicapped and 21 unaffected controls (Tordjman et al. 1995). This finding does not contradict the theory that sex hormones are associated with autism, as the study looked at postnatal hormone levels rather than prenatal levels, which would be more relevant to the shaping of brain development. There are no studies to date examining the relationship if any between FT levels and autism spectrum conditions.

Insel, O'Brien, and Leckman (1999) argue that three observations about autism are consistent with the idea that relevant neurobiological events take place early in the development of the central nervous system, and involve a cascade of complex gene-environment interactions. First, autism is, by definition, a developmental syndrome (DSM-IV), and its onset invariably occurs before the age of 3 years. Second, abnormalities in social interest can be observed even in the first few months of life (Lord 1995). Third, the existence of a sex bias is consistent with other neurodevelopmental disorders (Gillberg and Coleman 1992), and this lends further support to the role of the intra-uterine environment.

However, when considering the potential role of fetal testosterone in autism, it is important to keep in mind that many biological factors, both hormones and neurotransmitters, have been implicated in the condition. Two of the most prominent are oxytocin (Insel 1992, p. 315) and serotonin (Anderson, Horne, Chatterjee, and Cohen 1990; McBride et al. 1989; Tordjman et al. 1995). Gillberg and Coleman (1992) summarize a number of biochemical findings associated with autism. In addition to hyperserotonaemia, these include studies of catecholamine metabolism, cyclic AMP, amino acids, peptides, minerals, and ions, including evidence of increased lead levels in individuals with autism. Gillberg and Coleman also review some inconclusive evidence of immunological and thyroid dysfunction in autism. It could be that these different biological observations in patients with autism are all related in some way. For example, testosterone has been reported to affect the pattern of serotonin innervation in the hypothalamus (Simerly, Swanson, and Gorski 1985), and sex hormones have been observed to affect central serotonin metabolism (Biegon 1990). Testosterone was linked to immune functioning by Geschwind, who also suggested that the Y chromosome in the male affected the thyroid. It could be useful to look for links between the different theories (or parts of them) because they could all be relevant to explaining the biological causes of autism.

Why Do Sex Biases Occur?

In conditions where a sex bias exists, information regarding the origin of such a sex bias is essential in the understanding of the etiology of the condition. The existence of sex biases points to certain candidate mechanisms, such as genetics and hormones.

Skuse (2000) examines possible reasons for the sex difference in liability to autism. These include simple genetic models (which are not consistent with available data on the incidence of autism), X-linkage models (which have yielded no experimental support), a multifactorial liability threshold model, and a prenatal hormone model.

A multifactorial liability threshold model means that individuals can vary in the amount of genetic susceptibility they have for a disorder, and that there has to be a threshold amount of susceptibility in order for it to develop. It is suggested that females require a greater degree of genetic risk in order to develop autism. If this were the case, one would expect an excess of affected relatives in families of female probands. For autism, family data are not consistent with such a model.

A prenatal hormone model is one in which early levels of sex hormones are said to cause autism, presumably in genetically susceptible individuals. Skuse argues that the model cannot account for the observed superiority of females with autism and their mothers on spatial tasks. In reality, data are not yet available to support or refute this claim, as no studies have looked at the role of prenatal hormones in the development of autism. In addition, there is only a small amount of data available on the role of prenatal hormones in the development of spatial ability. If females with autism experience anomalous hormone conditions prenatally, and if such factors are familial, the data on spatial skills in such females actually support the model, assuming spatial skills are influenced by prenatal hormones. Skuse also argues that there is no evidence that females with very high testosterone are susceptible to autism. One reason for this might be that high prenatal levels of sex hormones do not always coincide with genetic susceptibility to autism. Finally, Skuse argues that there is no evidence for elevated rates of autism in relatives of female probands. This is said to be a problem for the prenatal hormone model because female probands should be at a greater genetic risk than males. Again, one explanation could be that the model relies on genetic liability's coinciding with an anomalous hormonal environment, which will not always happen.

Skuse's work on Turner's Syndrome may provide some insight into why certain developmental disorders are more common in males than in females. Turner's Syndrome affects females only, and is characterized by an incomplete or absent second X chromosome. Of interest here are Turner's Syndrome females with only one X chromosome, which can be either maternal (Xm, in 70 percent of cases) or paternal (Xp, in 30 percent of cases) in origin. Skuse compared Xm females to Xp females and found that Xp children displayed more social-cognitive dysfunction than Xm children did. This result is consistent with the hypothesis that there is an imprinted locus* on the X chromosome that influences the development of social-cognitive skills. If the hypothesized locus only expresses genes from the paternally derived X chromosome (Xp), we would expect normal females (karyotype 46 XmXp) to do better than

---

*This means that gene expression is dependent on which parent the gene came from.

normal males (karyotype 46 XmYp) on tests of social-cognitive function. In normal males, the X chromosome is maternally derived, so the genetic locus would be silenced. In normal females, one X chromosome is derived from each parent, so the locus would be expressed in at least half of the bodily cells (Skuse et al. 1997).

Skuse hypothesizes that social-communicative skills are due to the action of the imprinted locus. A predisposition to autism (due, perhaps, to low IQ, or to damage to the locus in females) impairs these skills. For a given cognitive domain, females are better than males, because males lack the imprinted locus. The same genetic liability to autism is worse for males than for females, because the male is already disadvantaged in that domain (Skuse 2000).

Support for the imprinted X chromosome theory comes from a study by Creswell and Skuse (1999) that linked Turner's Syndrome to autism for the first time. Ten out of 221 girls (4.5 percent) with Turner's Syndrome were found to have autism. Each of these 10 girls had a normal Xm and missing or abnormal Xp. Proportionately, 10 out 156 (6.4 percent) Turner's Syndrome females with a missing or abnormal Xp were found to be autistic. Zero out of 65 with an intact Xp were affected. One fact requiring explanation is that normal males also lack Xp, but their rate of autism is not as high as in the Turner's Syndrome females with a missing or abnormal Xp.

Another condition which is more common in males than females is language delay. Tallal, Ross, and Curtiss (1989) carried out an analysis of families of 62 language-impaired probands. The study revealed that affected mothers gave birth to a disproportionately high number of sons, whereas affected fathers had equal numbers of sons and daughters. Male and female children of affected parents were equally likely to be affected themselves, but the high number of sons born to affected mothers gave rise to the male-biased sex ratio, in cases among the offspring. Examination of probands who did not have an affected parent failed to reveal a male-biased sex ratio.

Perhaps affected mothers were more likely to conceive sons, because of the likelihood that a child of theirs would inherit their language problems. Such problems could possibly be more disadvantageous to a girl (in evolutionary terms) because females rely more heavily on their social-communicative skills than males do. A male child could be less disadvantaged by language impairment and could be more likely to lead a normal life and successfully reproduce. This reasoning is based on the writing of Matt Ridley in *The Red Queen* (1993). Ridley describes the observation that 60 percent of the children born to American presidents have been male—a significant deviation from the expected 50:50 male:female ratio. He also gives other examples of biased sex ratios in groups of humans and animals that are in "good condition." Using the work of Trivers and Willard (1973), Ridley outlines the argument that in certain cultures, at certain times in history, it would have been adaptive for highly privileged families to have sons, who could inherit their wealth and status. Poorer families would have benefited from having girls, because they could marry into richer families.

Tallal (1991) cites evidence that increased male births are associated with maternal stress and abnormal levels of sex hormones, especially testosterone (James 1986). Maternal gonadotrophin levels are said to influence the sex of the zygote, high levels being associated with the production of girls. It is also suggested that high levels of testosterone might be associated with production of boys, but no mechanism is proposed (James 1983). Tallal also cites a small amount of circumstantial evidence that stressful occupations, androgen levels, and sex ratios are linked. Women in stressful occupations are reported to have higher androgen levels than those in less stressful occupations, and stress is associated with reduced testosterone levels in men. Men with increased stress father more girls (Purifoy and Koopmans 1979; Kreuz, Rose, and Jennings 1972).

There are some conditions that are more prevalent in females than in males, and there is some evidence for a hormonal role in them. Among these conditions are the affective and anxiety disorders, including depression (Rubin 1981; Tallal 1991; Weissman et al. 1988; Geschwind and Behan 1982). Comparisons of plasma testosterone levels in males with depression to controls have been made (Rubinow and Schmidt 1996). Some studies report no difference (Davies et al. 1992); some others have found higher testosterone levels in controls (Rubin 1981). One study found a negative correlation between testosterone level and severity of depression (Davies et al. 1992).

Additionally, Berenbaum and Denburg (1995) cite an observation by Rose and Mackay (1985) that most multi-system autoimmune diseases occur predominantly in women. Examples include systematic lupus erythematosus, multiple sclerosis, myasthenia gravis, thyroid disease, arthritis, and some allergies. Geschwind argued that such conditions were predominant in young women in whom testosterone effects were at a minimum and this fitted the increased prevalence in males with age. Another condition likely to be influenced by hormones is Alzheimer's disease, which is also is more common in females. Estrogen-replacement therapy might help to slow down the disease (McEwen 1994).

A further possible explanation for the increased prevalence of developmental disorders in males is concerned with the way in which the brain recovers from early damage. De Courten-Myers (1999) argues that if overproduction of neurons can compensate for damage, the magnitude of overproduction may be related to the amount of protection offered. Male fetuses appear to overproduce neurons to a lesser extent than females. This might explain greater developmental problems in boys, resulting from early brain damage. On the other hand, adult women have a lower number of cortical neurons than men, and a greater number of neuronal processes. This means that there is a greater loss of connections per neuron lost, and it might explain why women suffer more from dementia in later life.

It is likely that a range of factors contribute to sex biases in disorders, not just hormonal ones. Shaywitz, Shaywitz, Fletcher, and Escobar (1990) argue that the high number of males with diagnosed reading disability could be due to referral bias, because of increased activity level and disruptive behavior in those boys.

Nevertheless, the study of disorders of sexual development and of sex bias in disorders provides further clues that fetal testosterone can affect subsequent brain development. In the next chapter we will put this in context by considering the range of research strategies available for investigating this question.

5

Research Strategies for Studying Hormone Effects

The traditional approach to studying hormone-behavior relations in humans has been to examine if hormonal fluctuations in adulthood have transitory effects on cognition. For example, there is some evidence that spatial ability in men is partly dependent on short-term variations in androgen levels. The effects of circulating hormones are superimposed on changes induced prenatally. Hampson and Moffat (1994) cite two studies that associate increased testosterone with reduced spatial performance both diurnally (Mackenberg, Broverman, Vogel, and Klaiber 1974) and seasonally (Kimura and Hampson 1994). Evidence suggests that, in the Northern Hemisphere at least, mean testosterone levels are higher in autumn than in spring. This is probably related to the optimal time for mating. Seasonal variations have been found in spatial performance, performance being better in spring than in autumn (Kimura and Toussaint 1991).

There is also evidence that hormonal fluctuations of the menstrual cycle in women can affect cognition. The midluteal phase of the menstrual cycle (between ovulation and menstruation) is characterized by high estrogen and progesterone, and the late menstrual phase is characterized by low levels of these hormones. In the midluteal phase, relative to the late menstrual phase, women were better at female tasks (manual dexterity) and poor on a male-type perceptual-spatial test. These results were supported in a second experiment using a wider battery of sexually dimorphic tests (Hampson and Kimura 1988). However, estrogen and progesterone levels vary in parallel during those two phases, which makes it impossible to separate the effects of the two hormones. Hampson (1990) compared performance during the menstrual phase against performance 1 or 2 days before ovulation, when there is a surge in estrogen but no surge in progesterone. Again high estrogen was associated with enhanced performance on female tasks and with impaired performance on male tasks. The study also revealed enhanced right-ear superiority on a dichotic listening task during the high-estrogen phase. In the rat, there is evidence that the brain (e.g., the hippocampus) is affected by hormonal variations of the reproductive cycle (McEwen 1994).

Correlational Studies

Correlational studies carried out to date on the effects of sex hormones on behavior and cognition fall into three main categories according to how the hormone data were collected. A few studies have looked at hormone levels in amniotic fluid, others at levels in cord blood at birth, and others at salivary or serum levels in adults.

Amniocentesis
One research group conducted a longitudinal study of children whose mothers had undergone amniocentesis. They were able to analyze the amniotic fluid thus obtained for hormone levels.

The following three experiments formed part of the longitudinal study.

Finegan, Niccols, and Sitarenios (1992) observed 30 girls and 30 boys at 4 years of age. In girls, language comprehension and conceptual grouping were quadratically and inversely related to fetal testosterone (inverse U-shaped curve). There was also a inverse linear relationship to counting and sorting and numerical ability. In boys, there were no significant correlations between FT levels and outcome measures. This study tested for FT correlations with a wide range of cognitive tasks. Although Finegan et al. acknowledge that it would be better to specifically use sexually dimorphic tests, they argue that such tests were not available for the age group studied. However, there does not seem to be a strong motivation for employing the particular tasks that they used, and the study appears to be a fairly general search for FT correlates.

A further stage of the longitudinal study was carried out by Grimshaw, Sitarenios, and Finegan (1995b). This was a study of sixty 7-year-old children whose mothers had undergone amniocentesis. The test of most interest here involved mental rotation, which is known to yield reliable sex differences. A positive correlation between rotation rate and fetal testosterone was observed for girls. Findings were non-significant for boys but seemed to be in the opposite direction. Looking at both boys and girls together, the results could be described as quadratic (i.e., an inverse U shape). One problem with this study was that a number of children were excluded from the final analysis. Only 21 girls and 20 boys met criteria in the training phases, and these were further reduced to 12 girls and 13 boys, who were judged to have used a rotational strategy (i.e., their response time correlated to the angle through which they had to mentally rotate). These results do fit the Geschwind Hypothesis. The quadratic curve means that there is an optimum level of fetal testosterone for spatial performance in the low male range. This predicts that males will be advantaged at spatial performance and that there will be more males in the very high and very low ranges of spatial performance. The FT levels of females will generally not get high enough for there to be a detrimental effect on spatial performance.

The study group was assessed again at 10 years of age. Grimshaw et al. (1995a) included 25 girls and 28 boys in a study that examined handedness and performance on a dichotic words test and an emotional words test. In girls, increased fetal testosterone was associated with increased right-handedness and increased left-hemisphere language. In boys, increased fetal testosterone was related to increased right-hemisphere representation of affect. The results in boys support the Callosal Hypothesis in that increased testosterone is associated with increased lateralization. The Callosal Hypothesis did not, however, comment on girls. The results do not fit the Geschwind Hypothesis, because here increased fetal testosterone is associated with more typical patterns of asymmetry. The observation of different patterns in boys and girls was not thought to be problematic. It was argued that testosterone levels might be more reliable in one sex and that critical periods might be different in each sex. Additionally, one point in time might represent left-hemisphere development in one sex and right-hemisphere development in the other. The study reported that there was no effect of birth stress and that parental handedness was related to lateralization. Parental handedness and hormones contributed differently to the variance in the outcome data, which suggested that genetic effects are not manifested via hormonal mechanisms.

Umbilical-Cord Blood

Jacklin, Wilcox, and Maccoby (1988) measured five steroid hormones including testosterone in umbilical-cord blood at birth. In females, testosterone was inversely correlated with spatial ability at 6 years, but there was no correlation in boys. Trends for boys and girls were in the opposite direction to each other for testosterone, estradiol, and progesterone. The testosterone result in females was the opposite direction to that predicted by Geschwind. In an earlier study, testosterone, estradiol, and progesterone were measured in cord blood and found to be significantly correlated to timidity later in life in boys but not in girls (Jacklin, Maccoby, and Doering 1983). Studies have generally not found sex differences in hormone levels in cord blood at term (Maccoby, Doering, Jacklin, and Kraemer 1979), so this might not be the best time to look for hormone correlates for sexually dimorphic behaviors.

Salivary Testosterone

Gouchie and Kimura (1991) divided men and women into groups according to whether they had high or low salivary testosterone. Men with lower testosterone (below the median) performed better than other groups (above the median) on spatial and mathematical tasks. Women with high salivary testosterone scores did better than other women on the same measures. No significant relationships were found for female-typical tasks. Moffat and Hampson (1996) found an inverse U-shaped relationship between spatial ability and salivary testosterone in right-handers but not left-handers. They concluded that hand preference might mediate the observed effects.

Adult Serum

With regard to adult serum testosterone levels, Christiansen and Knussmann (1987b) found that testosterone in men was positively correlated with measures of spatial ability and field independence and negatively correlated with measures of verbal production. Serum and salivary androgens in adult men were also observed to be related to self-reported spontaneous aggression (Christiansen and Knussmann 1987a). Knussmann, Christiansen, and Couwenbergs (1986) found a positive correlation between serum testosterone and sexual activity in men.

All the reviewed research strategies have provided important information on the relationship of testosterone to cognition and behavior, but the only one that can inform us about the role of *fetal* testosterone on later brain, cognitive, and behavioral development is amniocentesis. In the remainder of this book we describe our own recent studies of such "amniocentesized" children.

6

"Amniocentesized Children": From Fetus to 12 Months

Measuring Fetal Hormone Levels

Finegan, Bartleman, and Wong (1991) proposed that amniotic fluid obtained for routine amniocentesis during pregnancy could be assayed for fetal hormone levels, during the period that is important for sexual differentiation of the brain, allowing the study of the importance of these hormones on postnatal development.

During early pregnancy, fetal testosterone is thought to enter the amniotic fluid by means of diffusion through the fetal skin; later it enters the fluid via fetal urine (Robinson, Judd, Young, Jones, and Yen 1977). Dörner (1976) was the first to note that levels of testosterone in amniotic fluid reflect those in fetal circulation, and that they are therefore a marker of fetal exposure. The validity of the suggested technique depends on a strong correlation between hormone levels in amniotic fluid and actual fetal levels. Data on the degree of correlation are not available, but it is believed to be high. Furthermore, amniotic-fluid levels of testosterone are found not to correlate with maternal levels (Rodeck, Gill, Rosenberg, and Collins 1985). This implies that amniotic-fluid levels reflect the fetal rather than the maternal contribution to amniotic-fluid testosterone levels (Dawood and Saxena 1977). Abramovich et al. (1987) found that the ratio between testosterone and follicle stimulating hormone could be used to a high degree of accuracy to predict the sex of 14 twin pairs in separate amniotic sacs. This showed that amniotic fluid could be a good source of information on the fetus.

Levels of fetal testosterone vary greatly during gestation. In the male, they vary from undetectable to near adult levels. Studies reveal that the greatest sex differences in FT levels are generally detectable around weeks 14–16 in fetal serum (Nagamani, McDonough, Ellegood, and Mahesh 1979; Abramovich 1974). Levels begin to decline at 17 weeks and continue to decline until term, when there is no real sex difference. In amniotic fluid, maximal sex differences have been measured between week 12 and week 18 (Nagamani et al. 1979; Rodeck et al. 1985).

Sexual differentiation of the brain is thought to take place between week 14 and week 18—that is, during the period of high plasma testosterone in the male fetus, and during and after the differentiation of the genitalia. This idea has been supported by studies of the uptake of labeled testosterone by aborted fetuses (Abramovich and Rowe 1973). However, contradictory evidence was reported when a study of mid-trimester fetal brains failed to reveal estrogen, androgen, or progestin receptors (Abramovich, Davidson, Longstaff, and Pearson 1987).

Prenatal Hormones and the Features of Autism: Social and Language Development

One interesting area to investigate is the relationship between prenatal hormones and the development of autism spectrum conditions. These conditions are from 4 times to 9 times more common in males and may represent an extreme form of the "male brain." However, autism is relatively rare, affecting only one in 200 births (Gillberg and Wing 1999), so this would require a large sample. The same argument applies to developmental language delay, which is also relatively rare (approximately 3 percent of children).

An alternative approach to studying disorders is to examine the normal development of behaviors known to be disrupted in certain disorders. This approach furthers the understanding of those behaviors, as well as guiding predictions for clinical research.

In our own studies (Lutchmaya et al. 2002; Knickmeyer et al. 2003), we examined the relationships between FT levels and behaviors that are impaired in autism. We pursued this line of examination because of the theoretical arguments linking autism, FT, and maleness, as well as the documentation of sex differences in those domains. Sexual dimorphism suggests that sex hormones might play a role in the development of a characteristic. The domains we examined were social and communicative development. The study was longitudinal in design. FT data were obtained during pregnancy, and each child was followed up at three different time points.

Time Scale of Our Study

The design of our study incorporated measurements spanning up to 30 months for each subject (table 6.1). We took advantage of the fact that at at Addenbrooke's Hospital in Cambridge samples of amniotic fluid are kept in frozen storage

Table 6.1
Time scale of study.

Time point	Cumulative time	Event	Contact with children
Time 0	0 months	Mother undergoes amniocentesis	None
Time 1	Approx. 6 months*	Birth of child	None
Time 2	18 months	Child turns 12 months of age	First contact made here
Time 3	24 months	Child turns 18 months of age; amniotic fluid discarded by hospital	Second contact 6 months later
Time 4	30 months	Child turns 24 months of age	Third contact 12 months after initial contact

*Time between amniocentesis and birth.

until around 18 months after the birth of the child. This allowed contact to be first established with children at Time 2, reducing the time span of study for each subject to 12 months, while still allowing retrospective access to data relating to Time 0.

The availability of patients who had undergone amniocentesis was established during discussions with the relevant laboratories at Addenbrooke's Hospital. The labs analyze samples of amniotic fluid for a number of hospitals in East Anglia. Approximately 1,000 samples are analyzed per year. To facilitate the administrative side of the project, recruitment of participants was attempted at only four hospitals. We estimated that the number of patients from these four hospitals would total 600 per year.

Predictor Variables

The main predictor variables of interest are sex and FT level. We also included a range of control variables which were thought to have some influence on the outcome measures in the study. The control variables were amniotic-fluid estradiol level, amniotic-fluid AFP level, number of siblings, age of parents, and educational level of parents.

Estradiol was included for a number of reasons. It is the most biologically active estrogen. It may have both feminizing and masculinizing effects on development. Because of its feminizing effects, estradiol could be considered as an opposing force to testosterone. It is also made from testosterone (via aromatization), which suggests that levels of the hormones are related. In rodent models testosterone is known to exert its masculinizing effects by first being converted to estradiol in the brain, so it is important to consider estradiol when looking at the biological activity of testosterone. Owing to the relationship between testosterone and estradiol, and owing to the complex effects of estradiol, it is difficult to predict what the effects of amniotic-fluid estradiol levels on development should be. Alpha-fetoprotein was included because it is said to be a general marker of fetal health and because it may be an important binding protein in amniotic fluid. This is of relevance, because it is the unbound testosterone that is of greatest biological interest.

The remaining variables (number of siblings, parents' age, and parents' education level) were included because they were thought to be highly significant factors in the social environment of the child, and could therefore have an important influence on child development. These factors could potentially influence the amount and nature of interaction between children, their parents, and their peers. The influence of parents' education on developmental outcome is supported by two recent studies that report a relationship between mother's education level and language and cognition in children (Dollaghan et al. 1999; Lyytinen, Laakso, Poikkeus, and Rita 1999).

Parents' education level was measured by classifying parents on a five-point scale: 1 = no formal qualifications, 2 = "O" level, General Certificate of Secondary Education or equivalent (which equates to high school graduation in the US), 3 = "A" level, Higher National Diploma or vocational qualification (which equates to specialist training in the US), 4 = university degree, 5 = postgraduate qualification. The scores for both parents were added together.

Ethical Issues

As the potential participants in this study were recruited from the time they were hospital patients, approval was required for the study from the relevant hospital Local Research Ethics Committees (LRECs). This was essential, as issues surrounding pregnancy and child development are highly sensitive, and as the target families had all experienced amniocentesis, we viewed them as a particularly sensitive group.

The following considerations were of prime importance to us. First, we did not want to contact anyone inappropriately— for example, anyone who had undergone amniocentesis and then gone on to have a miscarriage or termination. One recent study reported the rate of fetal loss following amniocentesis as being between 1.1 percent and 3 percent (Saltvedt and Almstrom 1999). It was therefore necessary to devise a screening method that would allow us to exclude families where necessary. We chose to use a two-stage method for this screening process. In the first instance, medical records were examined for evidence that a family should not be contacted. General Practitioners were then asked to give permission for us to contact their patients.

A second major area of concern was ensuring that we approached potential children in such a way that the minimum upset and anxiety would be caused. We identified the following potential areas of sensitivity. Families would be contacted by a researcher regarding a medical matter, which they might have felt was private between themselves and their doctor, so might consider this as a breach of doctor patient confidentiality. We would be reminding families of the amniocentesis, which they had experienced up to 18 months earlier. This was potentially a highly upsetting time for those involved. Finally, the idea of their child undergoing tests or assessments could be worrying to some families.

We tackled these issues as follows. In the initial letter, we approached the subject of amniocentesis with caution, acknowledging that this may have caused anxiety and emphasizing that we did not wish to cause any further anxiety. Feedback from mothers later indicated that some of them could see how our motives were to be as careful as possible to avoid distress, but that this may have been excessive for some mothers who had found the procedure less difficult. Nevertheless, our letter was designed to avoid upsetting even one patient, even if such patients were in a minority. The letter reassured mothers that the study would not involve any further medical procedures, that all assessments would be non-invasive and non-intrusive and that all information would be treated in the strictest confidence. If mothers did not return their consent form, recruitment was not pursued.

All procedures and documents were approved by the relevant LRECS. To avoid breaching doctor-patient confidentiality, all patients were contacted by a hospital consultant.

Recruitment of Children

Stage 1: Screening of Medical Records

Medical records of 500 patients were screened. These patients were women who had undergone routine amniocentesis between June 1996 and June 1997 and whose babies were due between January and December 1997.

Children were excluded at this stage according to the following criteria. These criteria were formulated to include suitable children while avoiding contacting anyone inappropriately or introducing potential confounding variables (e.g., twinning).

Exclusion Criteria at Stage 1

- Amniocentesis revealed a chromosomal abnormality.
- Pregnancy ended in miscarriage or termination.
- Child suffered neonatal or infant death.
- Child suffered significant medical problems after birth.
- Twin pregnancy.
- Exceptional circumstances indicated that contact would not be appropriate—e.g., maternal illness, child in care, previous amniocentesis revealing abnormality.
- Medical records were not located.

If children were not excluded at this stage, the following data were collected from their medical records:

- confirmation of name, address, and date of birth of mother
- name, date of birth, and sex of child
- gestational age at amniocentesis
- gestational age at birth
- name and address of General Practitioner.

Of the 500 patients whose records were screened, approximately 400 were included and 100 were excluded, according to the above criteria.

Stage 2: Obtaining Consent from General Practitioners

If a child was not excluded during Stage 1, a letter was sent to the GP. This letter briefly explained the study and asked the GP to return a consent form indicating whether or not the GP consented to our contacting the patient. Stage 2 was included because it was thought that GPs would have more up-to-date information on their patients than was available in their obstetric files, and that they would have insight into whether it would be appropriate to contact them. GPs were not asked to give a reason if they withheld consent. In a number of cases, they were able to inform us that the patient had moved away and to provide the new address if known. GPs were typically contacted 4–6 weeks before any planned contact with the patient.

Approximately 400 GPs were contacted; 250 gave consent, and 150 either withheld consent, did not reply, or informed us that the patient was no longer registered with them. In such cases, GPs were unable to provide us with details of the patient's new GP.

Stage 3: Contacting Patients

If during Stage 2 a GP gave consent for a patient to be contacted, that patient was sent a letter inviting her to take part in the study. If a mother wished to participate, she was asked to return a consent form in a postage-paid envelope. If a mother did not reply, no further attempt was made to contact her.

Measurement of Fetal Testosterone

Assays were carried out by the Department of Clinical Biochemistry at Addenbrooke's Hospital. Amniotic fluid was extracted with diethyl ether. Recovery experiments have demonstrated 95 percent recovery of testosterone via this method. The ether was evaporated to dryness at room temperature, and the extracted material was redissolved in assay buffer. The testosterone was assayed by the DPC "Count-a-Coat" method (Diagnostic Products Corp., Los Angeles, CA 90045-5597), which uses an antibody to testosterone coated onto propylene tubes and a 125-I labeled testosterone analogue. The detection limit of the assay is approximately 0.1 nmol/l. This method measures total extractable testosterone, not just free unbound testosterone. AFP and estradiol levels were also measured by the same lab.

Follow-up at 12 Months

Parents were invited to bring their 12-month-old infants to the study, via the recruitment procedure described above. All infants were accompanied by their mothers, with the exception of four who were accompanied by their fathers. Figure 6.1

shows the layout of the testing room used for this study. The infant, the parent, and a female experimenter (SL) were filmed for approximately 20 minutes during free play.

Toys were presented in random order. When one toy was presented, the preceding one was removed. The parents were told that we were interested in the child's natural reactions and so they should not try to steer the child's play behavior too much. They were instructed to react to the child as they normally would, if the child approached them. This allowed us to measure behaviors initiated mainly by the child, without creating an unnecessarily strange environment for them. The child was placed on the play mat and was free to move around. The parent was asked to try and keep the child within the field of view of the video camera (i.e., on the mat) as much as possible.

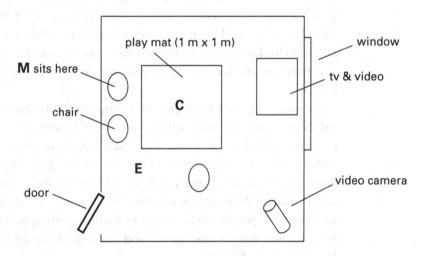

Figure 6.1
Layout of room used to test infants at 12 months of age. E: experimenter. M: mother. C: child.

Eye Contact at 12 Months

When these "amniocentesized children" reached the age of 12 months, we examined the relationship between their fetal testosterone and their eye contact. Before revealing the results, let us take a small digression into why eye contact is of interest.

Eye contact and perception of gaze direction have a number of functions. Social contact, for example, often depends initially on establishing eye contact with the social partner (Kawashima et al. 1999). Perception of gaze direction is important for decoding emotional expressions and mental states, and for orienting attention to interesting features of the environment.

For this experiment, eye contact was selected as a marker of social development at 12 months of age. The ability to engage in eye contact is considered to be a crucial stage in normal social development (Baron-Cohen 1995; Trevarthen 1979; Stern 1977). Studies have illustrated the importance of the eyes as a stimulus for very young infants, the abnormal use of gaze in autism and delayed social development in congenitally blind babies.

Evidence suggests that the eyes are an important stimulus for babies, even at a very early age. Maurer and Salapatek (1976) reported that infants as young as 2 months spent more time looking at the eye region than at any other part of the face. Stern (1977) observed that babies spend most of their time when awake in the feeding position looking at the faces of their mothers. It is possible that the infant feeding position is the basis for the role of gaze in the social world of the infant (Argyle and Cook 1976).

Findings in the autism literature also led to the selection of eye contact as a marker of social development. A number of studies have described either reduced or abnormal use of eye contact in autistic children (Swettenham et al. 1998; Phillips, Baron-Cohen, and Rutter 1992; Baron-Cohen 1989; Sigman, Mundy, Sherman, and Ungerer 1986; Mirenda, Donnelan, and Yoder 1983; Langdell 1978). The unusual eye-contact behavior observed in autism is thought to be quite specific and not simply due to a general deficit in face processing. Individuals with autism have demonstrated the ability to identify gender from the face alone (Baron-Cohen 1991) and to recognize simple emotions from the face (Baron-Cohen, Spitz, and Cross 1993). The specific abnormality in gaze behavior from an early age may help to explain the development of the condition, in which social impairment is a symptom (Baron-Cohen 1995).

Congenitally blind children, who obviously lack eye contact, can show delayed social development. This is discussed by Hobson (1993) who also reports increased autistic-like features in a group of congenitally blind children compared to sighted controls (Brown, Hobson, Lee, and Stevenson 1997). Such evidence suggests that normal social development is disrupted when the input normally gained via sight is lost.

Factors That Influence Use of Eye Contact

The way in which we use eye contact is determined by a range of factors (Kleinke 1986). These include personal factors (such as sex and age), experiential factors (such as past behavioral consequences of eye contact), relational factors (such as mother to child), and situational factors (such as being with a group of strangers). Kleinke cites a number of studies (of both adults and children) which have found sex differences in eye contact, with females generally showing more gaze in social dyadic interactions than males (Argyle and Cook 1976). Sex differences have been reported in the situational use of eye contact, such as males using more than females when in a threatening situation. Benenson (1993) demonstrated that 4- and 5-year-old girls showed greater enjoyment of dyadic interactions with a puppet than did boys, as measured by eye contact and smiling. Additionally, Podrouzek and Furrow (1988) found that 24- to 30-month-old girls showed more eye contact than boys in a free play session with their mothers and an experimenter. Such extensive evidence for sexual dimorphism in the use of eye contact provides strong motivation for examining the relationship between eye contact and fetal testosterone.

Brain Mechanisms for Gaze Perception

Some recent studies have revealed the brain regions likely to be involved in the perception of gaze, both in monkeys and humans (Wicker, Michel, Henaff, and Decety 1998; Baron-Cohen 1995). Findings suggest that brain mechanisms have evolved, specifically for the processing of information from the eyes, as this is such an important function.

In monkeys, neural populations have been identified that are sensitive to gaze direction. These have been located in the superior temporal sulcus (STS) and in the amygdala (Brothers, Ring, and Kling 1990; Perrett et al. 1990; Perrett et al. 1985). Wicker (1998) cites evidence that human patients with temporal lobe or amygdala damage who are impaired on face identification have also been found to exhibit poor discrimination of gaze, as have monkeys with STS lesions (Young, Hellawel, Wal, and Johnson

1996; Campbell, Heywood, Cowey, Regard, and Landis 1990). One human study using functional neuroimaging found that the left amygdala plays a general role in the interpretation of eye gaze direction and that activity of the right amygdala increases when gaze is directed toward the subject (Kawashima et al. 1999). These findings suggest that the human amygdala plays a role in processing social information from the face. In their human study, Wicker et al. (1998) found that gaze perception is supported by a distributed cortical network, although the study did not identify regions specifically involved in eye contact. The role of the STS in the processing of eyes was supported. The study also supported the role of the parietal cortex in the attentional component of gaze perception.

Evidence suggests that autism might be associated with amygdala damage (Courchesne 1997). Baron-Cohen et al. (1999) found that control children were better than individuals with autism at a task, which required them to attribute a mental state to a person, based on information from their eye region alone. The use of functional magnetic-resonance imaging in this study revealed that success on the task was associated with activation of the superior temporal gyrus, of areas of the prefrontal cortex, and of the amygdala. The autistic children did not use the amygdala to carry out the task and relied more on temporal lobe regions, possibly to compensate for amygdala abnormality. The amygdala theory of autism is described in Baron-Cohen et al. 2000.

Measurement of Eye Contact

Observation of true eye contact (i.e., the moment when two people are looking at each other's eyes) would require special viewing conditions (Kleinke 1986; Argyle and Cook 1976). For this reason, we decided to take a simpler measure as a proxy for eye contact—i.e., any time when the child looked at the parent's face. This is referred to as "face gaze" in Kleinke's review of eye-contact research (Kleinke 1986), and it is described as an episode where one person's gaze is directed at another person's face, and possibly eyes. Such alternative measures are employed because it is difficult to differentiate between eye and face gaze in a naturalistic experimental setting. Most studies reporting eye-contact data rely on such proxy measures. Therefore, our study is comparable to other experiments in the field.

A further reason for measuring face gaze instead of mutual eye contact is that eye contact depends on the behavior of both interactants—that is, both members of the dyad have to make eye contact at the same time. So if we measured eye contact, we would be looking at the social behavior of the observed dyad. Face gaze by the child will of course be greatly influenced by the relationship with the person he or she is looking at. However, the *child* initiates face gaze, so it is less directly dependent on the dyad than eye contact is.

The Children

Seventy-one 12-month-old infants (41 boys and 30 girls) took part in the study of fetal testosterone and eye contact. None of the children had younger siblings. The age of the infants on the day of testing lay between 357 and 431 days (mean = 386.72 days, standard deviation = 17.71). There was no difference in age between the sexes, and the distribution of ages did not differ between the sexes.

Table 6.2
Descriptive data for the 71 children (of both sexes) who took part in our study of fetal testosterone and eye contact

	n^*	Range	Mean	S.D.
FT (nmol/l)	70	0.125–1.800	0.701	0.415
Estradiol level (pmol/l)	71	6.20–2630.00	922.12	399.99
AFP level (Jmol/l)	71	3.10–23.60	10.62	4.00
Gestational age at amniocentesis (weeks)	59	14.00–21.00	16.64	1.68
Number of siblings	68	0.00–3.00	1.01	0.97
Mother's age at child's birth	71	24.00–46.00	35.45	4.62
Father's age at child's birth	62	28.00–53.00	37.44	5.62
Level of education attained by parents	60	4.00–10.00	6.67	1.63

*Number of children for whom data were available.

The eye-contact measurements for our study were taken over the entire testing session. Frequency of eye contact between infant and parent and frequency of eye contact between infant and experimenter were measured over the whole session. An episode of eye contact was scored whenever the child looked at the face of the adult. The average rate of eye contact was calculated and converted to a frequency score representing a 20-minute period. In addition, the total duration of eye contact was timed with a manual stopwatch.

Results of Our Study of Fetal Testosterone and Eye Contact

Girls made significantly more eye contact with their parent than boys did. A significant quadratic relationship was found between eye contact and fetal testosterone when data from

Table 6.3
Descriptive data for the 41 boys who took part in our study of fetal testosterone and eye contact.

	n^*	Range	Mean	S.D.
FT (nmol/l)	41	0.125–1.800	0.943	0.365
Estradiol level (pmol/l)	41	432.00–2630.00	929.93	409.57
AFP level (Jmol/l)	41	3.10–20.20	10.24	3.77
Gestational age at amniocentesis (weeks)	33	14.00–21.00	17.00	1.79
Number of siblings	38	0.00–3.00	1.05	0.93
Mother's age at child's birth	41	24.00–46.00	34.66	5.20
Father's age at child's birth	34	28.00–52.00	36.82	5.82
Level of education attained by parents	33	4.00–10.00	6.76	1.70

*Number of children for whom data were available.

Table 6.4
Descriptive data for the 30 girls who took part in our study of fetal testosterone and eye contact.

	n^*	Range	Mean	S.D.
FT (nmol/l)	29	0.150–0.800	0.358	0.161
Estradiol level (pmol/l)	30	6.20–1950.00	911.44	393.19
AFP level (Jmol/l)	30	4.00–23.60	11.14	4.32
Gestational age at amniocentesis (weeks)	26	14.00–19.00	16.19	1.44
Number of siblings	30	0.00–3.00	0.967	1.03
Mother's age at child's birth	30	27.00–42.00	36.53	3.49
Father's age at child's birth	28	30.00–53.00	38.18	5.37
Level of education attained by parents	27	4.00–10.00	6.56	1.58

*Number of children for whom data were available.

both sexes were examined together and when data from the boys were examined alone, but not when data from the girls were examined alone.

Two independent judges, who were blind to the FT data, coded the videotapes of the testing sessions. The second judge examined 20 percent of the session for 20 percent of children. The eye-contact frequency ratings of the two judges were highly correlated ($r = 0.91$, $p = 0.00$). Girls (mean = 22.01) made significantly more eye contact with their parents over 20 minutes than did boys (mean = 16.09) ($t = -2.42$, degrees of freedom = 69, $p = 0.02$).

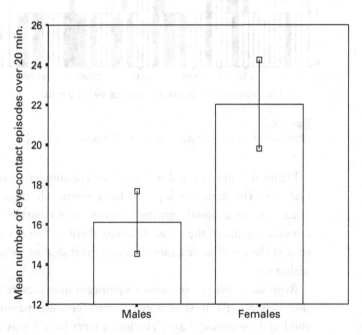

Figure 6.2
Mean frequency of eye contact for each sex. Error bars represent standard errors of mean.

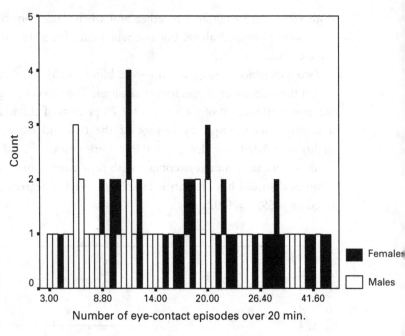

Figure 6.3
Distribution of eye-contact scores for each sex.

Figure 6.3 shows the distribution of eye-contact scores for each sex. The sexes overlap to a large extent, although there appears to be a slightly greater concentration of males at the low-scoring end of the scale. Although there is clear sex difference in the mean scores, there is also a great deal of variability within sex.

Regression analysis revealed a significant quadratic relationship between FT level and eye contact between parent and child at 12 months of age. The linear term for FT was also a significant inverse predictor of eye contact. Other biological

Table 6.5
Regression model. Dependent variable: ln(rate of eye contact per minute); $R^2 = 0.23$ (medium effect size); $F = 3.5$; $p = 0.04$; power > 0.88.

Model	β	Standard error	Significance
(Constant)	1.17	0.61	0.07
FT squared	2.29	0.90	0.02
FT	−4.10	1.54	0.01

and social factors were not found to have significant effects on eye contact over and above the effect of FT level and FT squared (table 6.5). The effects of FT and FT squared were also found to be significant when all seven predictors were present in the model. Further analysis reveals a significant quadratic relationship between FT level and eye contact between parent and child at 12 months of age for boys separately. The linear term for FT was also a significant inverse predictor of eye contact. The effects of FT were also found to be significant when all six predictors* were present in the model.

In summary, girls made significantly more eye contact with their parent than boys at 12 months of age. FT level was quadratically related to eye contact between a parent and 12-month-old infant. The linear term for FT was also a significant predictor of eye contact. This relationship was observed when data for both sexes were examined together and also when data for the boys was analyzed alone. No significant relationship was observed between FT level and eye contact for girls. In previous studies, Finegan, Niccols, and Sitarenios (1992)

---

*Sex was included as a predictor in the combined analysis but not in the within-sex analysis.

and Jacklin, Wilcox, and Maccoby (1988) reported significant findings for girls but not for boys.

The sex difference in eye contact was as we expected, given previous findings. Evolutionary theorists have characterized such sex differences as reflecting traditional sex roles (Kleinke 1986). Differential social influences on the sexes could also be involved. The present study reveals biological factors that can help explain the sex difference. The biological account is supported by the identification of possible brain regions involved in the processing of gaze.

When the data from both sexes were examined together, the quadratic term for FT was found to be a significant predictor of eye contact. It appeared that eye contact decreased with FT in the lower FT range, and the opposite was true in the higher FT range. The linear term for FT was also a significant predictor of eye contact: eye contact decreased with increasing levels of FT. One possible explanation for the quadratic finding was that the result was describing a sex difference. That is, one half of the quadratic graph represented the relationship between eye contact and FT within sex for girls and the other half represented the relationship within sex for boys.

The idea of a different relationship within sex was not completely unexpected. Grimshaw, Sitarenios, and Finegan (1995) described a positive correlation between FT and mental rotation at 7 years of age within girls, and the opposite pattern within boys. The resulting graph of FT against mental rotation ability (for both sexes together) was described as an inverted U shape. This meant that the optimum FT level for mental rotation ability lay in the low male range. As FT level increased in girls, their mental rotation ability increased. The FT level of girls is generally never high enough for there to be a detrimental effect on spatial ability, as was observed in boys, whose mental rotation score decreased with increasing FT level. The results obtained were said to fit the predictions of the Geschwind model (Finegan et al. 1992), as they accounted for males being generally better at spatial tasks than females. They also accounted for the observation that more males than females tend to show either very good or very poor spatial abilities.

As sex was discarded from the regression model, the effect of FT (and FT squared) appeared to be more important. However, in order to investigate fully whether the quadratic relationship observed in our study for both sexes together was simply describing a sex difference, it was necessary to remove sex as a variable and analyze the data within sex. The quadratic relationship was observed once again within boys. There was also an inverse relationship between eye contact and the linear term for FT level. The replication of the finding within sex for boys was critical, as it showed that there was a quadratic relationship between FT and eye contact that did not rely on sex.

One way to interpret this result from our eye-contact study would be as the opposite of the Grimshaw findings. Grimshaw et al. (1995) found an inverted-U-shaped relationship between FT and spatial ability, whereas here we have described an upright-U-shaped relationship between FT and social ability. At present, there are insufficient empirical grounds to assume that spatial and social ability are inversely related, and the observation of high frequencies of eye contact in the high and low FT ranges is not as readily explained as the equivalent finding for low levels of spatial ability. However, Baron-Cohen has argued that in autism deficits in empathizing may exist alongside superiority in systemizing (2002). This means that, if an individual is impaired in their empathizing (i.e., in understanding of the social world), that individual may spend more time interacting with the non-social world, thereby enhancing his understanding of it (i.e., his systemizing). Extended to non-clinical populations, such an argument could help account for an inverse relationship between social and spatial ability.

There are a number of possible explanations for the quadratic relationship observed in the data for the boys. There may be some threshold FT level at which the effect of FT on social development changes. That is, up to that threshold level an inverse relationship is observed, and above that level a positive correlation is observed due to some change in mechanism.

No significant relationships between FT and eye contact were observed for girls. This may be because there were only 30 girls in the sample, making the resulting model underpowered. A sample size of approximately 60 would be required to give the model a power of 0.80 assuming a similar effect size as was detected when both sexes were examined together. It would be necessary to run this experiment with a larger sample of girls before drawing any strong conclusions.

It could be that no relationship exists between fetal testosterone and eye contact for girls, or that an inverse linear relationship exists but not a quadratic one, due to the range of FT levels in girls. This could be because higher FT levels (normally observed in boys) are required for there to be a quadratic, or indeed any, relationship. It may be that different critical periods for brain development exist between the sexes (Goy and McEwen 1980) and that in girls the timing of the amniocentesis test is not optimal for the investigation of hormonal influences on social development. It has also been suggested that female fetuses are affected by stress more than male fetuses (Finegan et al. 1992), insofar as proportionally more of their FT is adrenal in origin. Although males do produce adrenal FT, the amount produced by the testes overshadows it, so the effects of stress on FT levels are less noticeable. Additionally, males and females may be affected differently by the various biological and non-biological factors considered in this experiment (or others beside these) and that different models of social development are appropriate for each sex.

In summary, fetal testosterone seems to be one contributing factor in determining amount of eye contact, producing not only the observed sex difference (a result in line with the only study of face perception in newborns (Connellan et al. 2001) but also a possible mechanism to account for individual differences in eye contact within each sex.

7

"Amniocentesized Children": From Fetus to 24 Months

Our second study was based on many of the same amniocentesized children as we met in the last chapter. We were interested in following them beyond their first birthday (the focus of the first study) to find out whether there are sex differences in language development at 18 and 24 months and to investigate the relationship between level of fetal testosterone and language development at these two ages.

To examine language development at 18 and 24 months, we used a Communicative Development Inventory (CDI) written by the Infant Development Group at Oxford University to assess vocabulary size in children between 12 and 24 months of age. The CDI is a checklist of 416 words divided into 19 categories, including animal names, body parts, quantifiers, and pronouns. Parents are instructed to mark each word their child can say.

The Oxford CDI is based on the American MacArthur CDIs, developed by Fenson et al. (1994). Fenson developed two vocabulary checklists—one for infants and one for toddlers—to assess communicative development in children. We chose to use the Oxford version in preference to the American version for two reasons. First, the Oxford version had replaced

American words with their British equivalents. Second, the Oxford version focused solely on single words, whereas the American version included gestures and early language structure. The Oxford version would allow us to look simply at single word vocabulary size, giving a simple numerical score for each child, suitable for our planned analysis.

Assessment of vocabulary size using the CDI relies solely on parental report. This technique carries a number of advantages. The parent observes the child in a wide range of contexts that are free from performance factors that might affect lab-based assessment. One study found that CDI scores for 20-month-olds correlated closely (0.60–0.80) to laboratory-based measures at 28 months, demonstrating that parental report could be a valid measure of language development in infants (Fenson et al. 1993). The method is also a highly time- and cost-effective way of gathering a large amount of data. In this case, families who had been unable to take part in other parts of the project due to practical constraints on visiting the lab were able to contribute data to Study C by post.

The Children Who Took Part in Our Study of Fetal Testosterone and Language

Our subjects ($n = 87$) were 18-month-old infants (40 girls, 47 boys). The descriptive data are summarized in tables 7.1–7.3. Sixty-one of the children had already taken part in our study at 12 months of age. Twenty-six joined at this stage, having been unable to take part in the eye-contact study for geographical or other practical reasons. One subject now had a younger sibling.

Table 7.1
Descriptive data for the 87 children (of both sexes) in our study of fetal testosterone and language.

	n^*	Range	Mean	S.D.
FT (nmol/l)	86	0.125–2.000	0.72	0.46
AFP level (Jmol/l)	87	1.90–23.60	10.89	4.18
Estradiol level (pmol/l)	86	404.00–2630.00	977.42	406.17
Gestational age at amniocentesis (weeks)	87	14.00–21.00	16.49	1.64
Mother's age at child's birth	87	23.00–46.00	35.36	4.78
Father's age at child's birth	66	26.00–53.00	37.17	5.73
Level of education attained by parents	87	4.00–10.00	6.62	1.66
Number of siblings	86	0.00–3.00	1.00	0.93
Age at which CDI data were collected (complete months)	86	17.00–20.00	17.61	0.71

*Number of children for whom data were available.

During the month in which the child was to turn 18 months of age, the parent was sent a copy of the Oxford CDI. The parents were instructed to indicate which of the words their child could say (out of a possible 416). They were asked to then return the inventory in a postage-paid envelope. The outcome measure was simply the child's score out of 416.

Parents were also asked to indicate which of the words their children could understand but could not yet say. This score was added to the number of words the child could say to give a total CDI score (i.e., total number of words the child could say or understand). The effect of the age (in months) at the time of data collection was also taken into account, as there was some

Table 7.2
Descriptive data for the 47 boys who took part in our study of fetal testosterone and language.

	n^*	Range	Mean	S.D.
FT (nmol/l)	47	0.125–2.000	1.01	0.43
AFP level (Jmol/l)	47	3.10–22.70	10.96	4.22
Estradiol level (pmol/l)	47	404.00–2630.00	979.40	430.01
Gestational age at amniocentesis (weeks)	38	14.00–21.00	16.53	1.83
Mother's age at child's birth	47	25.00–46.00	35.60	4.94
Father's age at child's birth	40	26.00–52.00	36.53	6.00
Level of education attained by parents	38	4 .00–10.00	6.68	1.76
Number of siblings	47	0.00–3.00	1.00	0.91
Age at which CDI data were collected (complete months)	46	17.00–19.00	17.50	0.66

*Number of children for whom data were available.

variation and it was thought that vocabulary might change quickly at this stage of development.

Results

Girls had a significantly higher vocabulary size than boys. A significant inverse relationship was found between fetal testosterone and vocabulary size with both sexes together, but not within either sex.

Girls (mean = 86.80) had a significantly higher vocabulary size than boys (mean = 41.77) (t = –2.79, d.f. = 80, p = 0.01)

In summary, this model shows that vocabulary size at 18 months was significantly related to sex, FT level, amniotic-

Table 7.3
Descriptive data for the 40 girls who took part in our study of fetal testosterone and language.

	n^*	Range	Mean	S.D.
FT (nmol/l)	39	0.150–0.800	0.38	0.16
AFP level (Jmol/l)	40	1.90–23.60	10.82	4.17
Estradiol level (pmol/l)	39	459.00–1950.00	975.03	381.01
Gestational age at amniocentesis (weeks)	35	14.00–21.00	16.46	1.44
Mother's age at child's birth	40	23.00–41.00	35.08	4.57
Father's age at child's birth	29	30.00–53.00	38.07	5.30
Level of education attained by parents	28	4.00–10.00	6.54	1.55
Number of siblings	40	0.00–3.00	1.00	0.96
Age at which CDI data were collected (complete months)	40	17.00–20.00	17.75	0.74

*Number of children for whom data were available.

fluid estradiol level, and parents' education level. The effects of FT and sex were also found to be significant when all eight predictors were present in the model.

This experiment found that, at 18 months, girls had a significantly larger vocabulary than boys. In addition, a significant inverse relationship was found between FT level and vocabulary size with both sexes together, but not within either sex.

When the data from both sexes were kept together, FT level was a significant predictor of vocabulary size. It is clear from figure 7.2 and table 7.4 that there is an inverse relationship between FT and vocabulary size. To further investigate the FT result, the analyses were repeated within sex. No significant

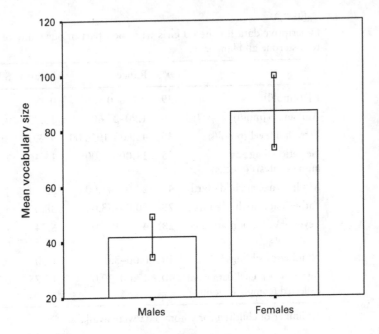

Figure 7.1
Mean vocabulary size for each sex at 18 months. Error bars represent standard errors of mean.

relationship was observed between FT level and vocabulary size within sex. This can be interpreted in a number of ways. One possible conclusion is that the significant FT result for both sexes together was simply describing a sex difference. However, the fact that both FT and sex were retained in the model suggests that FT has an independent effect on vocabulary size.

Inspection of the data suggests that an inverse relationship exists for the girls between FT and vocabulary size. With 40 girls in the sample, the analysis was sufficiently powerful to

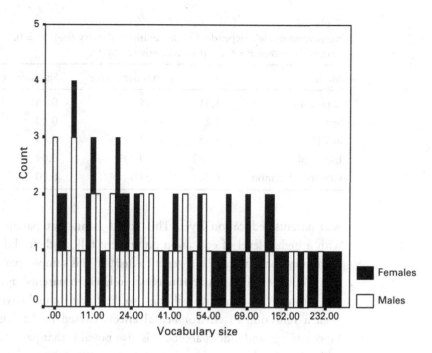

Figure 7.2
Distribution of vocabulary size scores for each sex at 18 months. There is some overlap between the sexes, although there is a greater concentration of females in the higher-scoring range and a greater concentration of males in the lower-scoring range.

detect a large effect size if a regression model was run and had four predictor variables (as with both sexes together). However, more children would be needed to detect a smaller effect size. Therefore, the lack of significant findings within sex (for boys and girls) may be related to low subject numbers.

When the data from both sexes were kept together, sex appeared to be the best predictor of vocabulary size (with girls scoring higher than boys). The next most significant predictor

Table 7.4

Regression model. Dependent variable: ln(vocabulary size); $R^2 = 0.25$ (large effect size); $F = 6.20$; $p = 0.00$; power > 0.99.

Model	β	Standard error	Significance
(constant)	1.31	0.85	0.13
Sex	1.25	0.36	0.00
ln(FT)	0.55	0.27	0.05
Estradiol	–0.00	0.00	0.04
Parents' education	0.22	0.08	0.00

was parents' education level. This could mean that parents with a higher level of education attainment talk to their children more, or that there is a genetic effect. In this sample, parents' education level was positively correlated to parents' age and indirectly to number of siblings, so the finding could have been a reflection of environmental effects caused by having more siblings and older parents. It is also possible that parents with a higher educational level score overestimated their child's vocabulary when completing the CDI. Estradiol level was an inverse predictor of vocabulary size. This fits with indications that estradiol can have masculinizing effects on development.

The biological result would undoubtedly be stronger if supported by a significant finding within sex. This would show that any FT effect persisted even when sex was no longer a variable, as in Experiment A1. However, it is not possible to draw strong conclusions until the within-sex findings are clarified by studies with greater numbers of participants.

In summary, our study of 18-month-olds shows a significant sex difference (female superiority) in vocabulary size. When a regression model was run, sex, the inverse linear term for fetal testosterone, parents' education level, and mother's age were all significant predictors of vocabulary size. Almost parallel results were also found at a later follow-up language study at 24 months of age (Lutchmaya et al. 2002). The subject numbers in this study were again similar to those in our study of eye contact at 12 months of age, so again lack of power may explain negative findings within sex.

The observed sex difference in vocabulary size (female superiority) is expected on the basis of previous studies. The sex difference may be mediated in part prenatally by the sex difference in FT level, or it may be due to sex differences in maturation rate. It may also be due to social factors, such as parents' talking more to girls than to boys, or to a combination of these factors. In the study described in chapter 6, we found that girls made more eye contact with their parents than did boys. If this finding indicates that girls generally spend more time in dyadic interactions, then they should experience more conversation and language learning as a consequence. One possibility is that the propensity of girls to engage in this dyadic interaction has its foundations in prenatal biology, and that, if parents are talking to girls more, it is because girls elicit this by their relative precocity of social-communicative development. This idea is supported by the biological findings of our experiment.

It would be useful to gain information about which specific parts of the brain support vocabulary learning, so that the plausibility of a fetal-hormone model can be assessed properly. One MRI study of boys with specific language impairment (SLI) failed to reveal any obvious lesions or abnormalities. It did, however, find consistent perisylvian abnormalities, and the authors argued that such a finding supported the role of prenatal alteration in brain development in the etiology of SLI (Plante, Swisher, Vance, and Rapcsak 1991). This supports the idea that prenatal factors are implicated in the development of language abilities in general.

It is, however, of great interest that the measure we have looked at yields a striking sex difference at two age points (18 and 24 months). A sex difference in vocabulary size is not usually thought to persist into adulthood. Adult females tend to have better verbal memory, spelling ability, and verbal fluency than adult males, though not larger vocabularies. The findings of this study raise two issues—why there is a sex difference in vocabulary size at 18 and 24 months of age and why in general females are superior to males at certain aspects of language.

So, just as in the last chapter, where we found that fetal testosterone predicted an aspect of social behavior at 12 months, here we find that fetal testosterone also predicts vocabulary development at 18 and 24 months. Whether these two findings are related or not remains to be fully understood.

8

"Amniocentesized Children": From Fetus to 48 Months

In our final follow-up (Knickmeyer et al. 2003), we saw 58 children (35 male, 23 female) aged 4.0– 4.25 years. We chose to study these children at age 4 because social cognition is rapidly developing at this point (Maccoby 1990, p. 298; Bartsch 1995, p. 374; Flavell 1993, p. 375). Our main measuring tool was the Children's Communication Checklist (Bishop 1998, p. 288).

The Children's Communication Checklist (CCC) consists of nine subscales. Scales A (speech) and B (syntax) measure traditional language skills. Scales C–G (inappropriate initiation, coherence, stereotyped conversation, use of context, rapport) are combined to make a single pragmatic language score. Scale H measures the quality of social relationships. Since syntactic aspects of language might benefit from either male-typical systemizing skills (Baron-Cohen 2002) or female-typical communication advantages, we did not expect a relationship with fetal testosterone in this area. Equally, since scales C–G cover a wide range of different skills, we did not expect any specific relationship with fetal testosterone. In contrast, we predicted that quality of social relationships (scale H) would be *inversely* related to testosterone. The checklist's designers included scale I, which measures restricted interests, to help determine whether a diagnosis of autism should be considered. Given that autism is characterized by social and theory of mind deficits, combined with restricted interests, we predicted that testosterone would be *directly* related to restricted interests. Mothers filled out the questionnaire.

Results showed that males had significantly higher FT levels ($t = -8.051$, $p < 0.00$, $d = 2.0$) and more restricted interests ($t = -2.371$, $p < 0.02$, $d = 0.68$). There was a trend for females to score better on quality of social relationships ($t = 1.743$, $p < 0.09$, $d = 0.47$).* The existence of sex differences on these scales indicates a possible role for FT. Bivariate (Pearson) correlations also suggested a relationship. For restricted interests, the correlation with FT was $r = 0.435$, significant at $p < 0.00$. For quality of social relationships, the correlation with FT was $r = -0.265$, significant at $p < 0.05$. Therefore, these scales were explored further.

Backward stepwise regression analyses showed FT to be the only significant predictor of both quality of social relationships and restricted interests. Table 8.5 shows the final regression model for quality of social relationships and restricted interests.

Child's sex was excluded as a predictor for both restricted interests and quality of social relationships while FT was retained in the model. This suggests that the sex differences seen in the scores are testosterone dependent. However, to further investigate whether the previous result might be due to a sex difference (not necessarily involving testosterone), we analyzed the relationship between these scores and FT within each sex using the same procedure described above. It should be kept in mind that this reduced the sample size by half and

*Here d is Cohen's d.

Table 8.1
Descriptive data for the children in the study of the role of fetal testosterone: scores on the Children's Communication Checklist. (Because the sample was small, parents' education was not used in later analyses.)

Variable	n^*	Range	Mean	S.D.
Fetal testosterone	58	0.13–1.80	0.79	0.46
Gestational age (weeks)	50	14–21	16.72	1.36
Alpha-fetoprotein (imol/l)	58	3.10–19.70	10.62	3.13
Estrogen (pmol/l)	57	404–2,630	962.35	427.31
Mother's age	57	23–43	35.02	4.64
Father's age	42	25–53	36.90	6.15
Parents' education	38	4–9	6.89	1.47
Number of siblings	54	0–3	1.1	0.96

*Number of children for whom data were available.

Table 8.2
Descriptive data for the 35 boys who took part in our FT-CCC study. (Because the sample was small, parents' education and parents' age were not used in later analyses.)

	n^*	Range	Mean	S.D.
FT (nmol/l)	35	0.13–1.80	1.02	0.39
AFP level (Jmol/l)	35	3.10–17.90	10.29	3.38
Estradiol level (pmol/l)	35	404.00–2,630.00	935.22	422.38
Gestational age (weeks)	28	14.00–21.00	16.86	1.65
Mother's age at child's birth	34	25–43	35.47	4.58
Father's age at child's birth	26	29–52	36.96	5.79
Parents' education	24	4–9	7.00	1.56
Number of siblings	31	0–3	1.10	1.01

*Number of children for whom data were available.

Table 8.3
Descriptive data for the 23 girls who took part in our FT-CCC study. (Because of the small sample, parents' education and parents' age were not used in later analyses.)

	n^*	Range	Mean	S.D.
FT (nmol/l)	23	0.17–0.80	0.40	0.19
AFP level (Jmol/l)	23	6.17–19.70	10.91	2.82
Estradiol level (pmol/l)	23	496–1,950	1,009.00	424.63
Gestational age (weeks)	22	14–19	16.61	1.11
Mother's age at child's birth	23	23–40	34.36	4.70
Father's age at child's birth	16	29–52	36.96	5.79
Parents' education	14	4–8	6.71	1.33
Number of siblings	23	0–3	1.09	0.92

*Number of children for whom data were available.

Table 8.4
Descriptive data for CCC scales showing a significant sex difference. (A higher score on the restricted interest scale indicates less restricted interests.)

	Quality of social relationships		Restricted interests	
	Boys	Girls	Boys	Girls
Mean	32.35	33	30.73	32.10
S.D.	1.66	1.00	2.30	1.70
Range	29–35	31–34	25–34	29–35
n	35	23	35	23

Table 8.5
Regression models. Restricted interests scores were reflected and logged before analysis. For quality of social relationships: $R^2 = 0.132$ (medium effect size), $F = 5.781$, $p = 0.021$, power > 0.60. For restricted interests: $R^2 = 0.182$ (medium effect size), $F = 11.133$, $p = 0.002$; power > 0.75.

Variable	Retained predictors	β	Standard error	Significance
Quality of social	Constant	33.576	0.424	
relationships	FT	–1.178	0.490	0.021
Restricted interests	Constant	0.475	0.052	
	FT	0.194	0.058	0.002

therefore reduced the power of the analysis. Data on father's age was unavailable for a number of cases, so we eliminated father's age from the within-sex comparisons in order to keep the sample as large as possible. Examination of univariate distributions showed that within girls, in contrast to the group as a whole and in contrast to boys, restricted-interest scores did not deviate from the Gaussian distribution. Therefore, untransformed versions of this variable were used when examining relations in girls. For quality of social relationships no significant relationship with FT was observed for boys or girls. For restricted interests, no relationship with FT was observed within girls. Within boys, FT was the only predictor retained in the model after the backward stepwise regression analysis.

Based on Geary's (1998) evolutionary model of sex differences in cognition, we initially predicted that girls would outperform boys on the CCC scales measuring quality of social relationships. A significant sex difference was confirmed for quality of social relationships, and this was related to FT levels in the group as a whole. We also predicted that boys would have more restricted interests than girls. A significant sex difference was confirmed, and this was related to FT in the group as a whole. An inverse relationship between restricted interests and fetal testosterone was also seen within boys when the sexes were examined separately.

Language ability did not show a significant sex difference. This is in keeping with Hyde and Linn's meta-analytic study of sex differences in verbal ability (Hyde 1988, p. 178). However, there are well-supported sex differences in some language measures, such as verbal fluency (Geary 1998, p. 358; Halpern 1992, p. 376). Also, as we saw in the last few chapters, our results showed that there are sex differences in vocabulary size at 12 months and 24 months, and that this is related to fetal testosterone (Lutchmaya et al. 2002, p. 268). The results from the CCC study suggest that gender differences in language occur only in some parts of the system.

In summary, the follow-up of these "amniocentesized" children shows a thread running through their development: fetal testosterone begins by affecting sociability (evident at 12 months as indexed by eye contact and face perception), later affects vocabulary (18 months and 24 months), and is still evident in shaping quality of social relationships at 48 months. The surprising result that fetal testosterone also influences restricted interests suggests that it may be involved in the development of autism, since that syndrome involves reduced sociability and very restricted interests.

Clearly, fetal testosterone may continue to show its effects beyond age 4, and it will be important to follow our children as they move through school and adolescence and into adulthood.

9

Limitations of the Reported Studies and Future Directions for Research

The biological limitations of the research reviewed above arise from the assumption that measurement of fetal testosterone in amniotic fluid informs us about FT levels at a time that is important for brain development. There is an additional assumption that influences on brain development at that time will be evident in the outcome measures we have reviewed. The amniocentesis test is carried out at a single variable time point (between weeks 14 and 22 in this sample), and we do not know how this time point relates to any sensitive periods for hormone influence on brain development. The sensitive periods may even differ between the sexes and according to which behavior is being studied.

For this sample, a relationship was observed within sex for girls between amniotic-fluid FT level and gestational age at amniocentesis. No such relationship was observed for both sexes together or within sex for boys. However, previous studies have reported that FT levels change quadratically (increasing and then declining) in male fetuses (Finegan, Niccols, and Sitarenios 1992). The availability of data on the matter is limited by the restricted availability of information from fetal serum and amniotic fluid. However, evidence suggests that the

FT level of the male begins to rise around week 8, peaking during week 16 and dropping again by week 24. There is no clear way of knowing how well the amniotic fluid obtained at a single time point within this period gives a true reflection of individual differences in serum FT level. For this sample, any variation of FT level over time was taken into account, so the variability of FT over gestation may not be a serious issue for the experiments reported here. With a big enough sample, it could be worth restricting the sample to "amnios" undertaken at a particular gestational age.

Another limitation of the biological model used here is that it does not take into account postnatal levels of testosterone. The second period of increased testosterone activity in the male (after the prenatal surge) occurs during the third month of life, and the testosterone levels at this time may play a role in sexual differentiation. It could be that the effects of this testosterone surge at 3 months are influenced by the FT levels experienced during the prenatal surge. If this were the case, then the relationships that we observed at 12 months of age and beyond would have been influenced.

It has been suggested that female fetuses are affected by stress more than male fetuses (Finegan et al. 1992), as proportionally more of their FT is adrenal in origin. Although males do produce adrenal FT, the amount produced by the testes overshadows it, so the effects of stress on FT levels are less noticeable. However, for the purposes of this project, it is the FT levels themselves that are of interest, not their origin.

A further issue, relating to the biological model constructed here, is that it relies on the measurement of whole FT present in the amniotic fluid. That is, any FT that is bound to other molecules is stripped from those binding agents and is measured along with the free FT. It might be that only free FT is relevant (as emphasized by Geschwind) if we are looking at biological activity. It could also be that other hormones need to be considered in order to refine the biological model. In order to explore the current model further, data from eye contact at 12 months were re-analyzed considering the ratio of FT to estradiol and the ratio of alpha-fetoprotein to FT. The estradiol:FT ratio was considered, to allow the balance between androgen and estrogen to be examined. This was done because the two hormones can be thought of as having opposing influences—i.e., masculinizing and feminizing. Supporting this model is the finding that the ratio of the lengths of the second and fourth digits (2D:4D), a sexually dimorphic trait thought to be fixed early in development, is related to the estradiol:FT ratio (Lutchmaya et al., in press). In addition, testosterone is a precursor to estradiol, so it is important to consider estradiol when looking at the biological activity of FT. The AFP:FT ratio was calculated because AFP may be the only significant binding protein in amniotic fluid, and unbound FT may be the most relevant when biological activity of FT is being considered. An additional source of error could be the technique used to analyze hormone levels in the amniotic fluid. However, this error should be fairly constant between subjects.

A further limitation of the study is that only children whose mothers had undergone amniocentesis could be included. This means that the parents involved in the study were typically of late parental age (because age is one indication for amniocentesis)—for example there were no parents in their teens or early twenties, and relatively few under 30. As well as being of late maternal age, a number of the mothers had other markers for

Down's Syndrome, such as those detected by the triple test,* and all underwent the stressful process of amniocentesis during pregnancy. It is also possible that certain social groups are underrepresented or overrepresented in those women who undergo amniocentesis. No British data on this aspect were readily available.

A direct consequence of using only children of mothers who had undergone amniocentesis was the limited available sample size. This meant that some of the experiments described were slightly underpowered, as was discussed in chapters 6 and 7.

One hypothesis that is consistent with these studies is that high prenatal testosterone levels are implicated in the development of autism and related conditions, but only in genetically susceptible individuals. This prenatal hormone model of autism is subject to criticisms, some of which are described in chapter 1. These include Skuse's argument that such a model cannot account for superiority on spatial tasks of females with autism or their mothers. In reality, data are not yet available to support or refute this claim, as no studies have looked at the role of prenatal hormones in the development of autism, and there is only a small amount of data available on the role of prenatal hormones in the development of spatial ability (Grimshaw, Sitarenios, and Finegan 1995). If females with autism do experience anomalous hormone conditions prenatally, and if such factors are familial, then the data on spatial skills in such females could be explained by the model, assuming that spatial skills are in fact influenced by prenatal hormones. Skuse also argues that there is no evidence that females

*The triple test is a form of maternal serum screening offered in the second trimester of pregnancy.

with very high testosterone are susceptible to autism. One reason for this might be that high levels of sex hormones prenatally do not always coincide with genetic susceptibility to autism. It is also not yet known if diagnosis of autism in males and females may be expressed differently, affecting ease of diagnosis in each sex. The data reported here show that high FT levels in either sex may in fact disrupt the development of behaviors important in autism.

Another potential problem for a prenatal hormone model of autism is that, if FT is involved in the etiology of autism, we might expect this to be reflected in the rate of autism in twins. As twins develop together in the womb, they should have a more similar prenatal hormone environment to each other than ordinary siblings would. This should be reflected in the degree of concordance for autism spectrum conditions between dizygotic twins. If the prenatal hormone environment is indeed crucial, then dizygotic twins should be more concordant for autism than other siblings (Skuse 2000).

It is likely that some inter-amniotic diffusion occurs in twin pregnancies (Henderson and Berenbaum 1997) and there is evidence from the animal literature that intrauterine position can affect sex-typical characteristics. For example, gerbils of either sex who developed between two males in utero have been found to show a more masculinized pattern of eye opening and paw use than controls (Clark, Robertson, and Galef 1993). There is also evidence for masculinization of female rats that were adjacent to male rats in utero (Hauser and Gandelman 1983, cited in Abeliovich, Leiberman, Teuerstein, and Levy 1984) and effects on estradiol level but not FT level in male mice that were adjacent to females in utero (Saal, Vom, Grant, McMullen, and Laves 1983).

One study of humans examined sex-typical play behavior in 35 girls with a male co-twin, in 36 girls with a female dizygotic twin, and in 20 girls with an older brother (Henderson and Berenbaum 1997). There was no evidence of masculinization of play preference in the girls with a male co-twin. This is in line with the idea that a mechanism is in place to protect female fetuses from excess androgen exposure (as in the female rat, where progesterone acts as an anti-androgen). A further study of handedness in opposite and same-sex twins found no association between sex of co-twin and handedness (Elkadi, Nicholls, and Clode 1999). This suggested that any effect of the co-twin on the hormonal environment was not sufficient to affect lateralization. However, one study did find evidence of increased spatial ability in girls with a male co-twin (Cole-Harding, Mostad, and Wilson 1988). Presumably this could also be due to the experience of having a male twin.

Current evidence suggests that dizygotic twins are no more concordant for autism than other siblings (Bolton et al. 1994). This does not necessarily contradict the theory that prenatal hormones and autism are linked. The intra-uterine environment might be similar enough from one pregnancy to another (within families) that the rate of autism is not different between twins and non-twin siblings. Additionally, even when FT levels are high, only genetically susceptible individuals should develop autism, and dizygotic twins would differ in their genetic susceptibility. A problem would exist if we suggested that prenatal hormones were the only mechanism for the development of autism. But clearly the strongest test of whether fetal testosterone is involved in autism would be a study of "amniocentesized" children who later develop autism. We are midway through such a study, and we await the results with interest.

Appendix

Information on Why These Mothers Opted for Amniocentesis

Some general information concerning the reason mothers underwent amniocentesis, their reaction to the amniocentesis, and the degree of obstetric complications reported is summarized here. Not all pregnant women undergo amniocentesis. Those who do have been identified (by a variety of means) as being at high risk of carrying a fetus with Down's Syndrome or other chromosomal abnormality. Mothers cited the following as the reasons for undergoing amniocentesis.

Results of Triple Test (60 Percent)

The triple test is a form of maternal serum screening offered in the second trimester of pregnancy. It is estimated that 85–95 percent of pregnant women in the Cambridge region opt to have this test. The levels of three substances made by the fetus and the placenta are measured in the maternal serum: human chorionic gonadotrophin (hcG),* unconjugated estriol, and

---

*Secretion of hcG begins very soon after implantation, and hcG is the substance commonly detected by pregnancy tests. It stimulates the biosynthesis of progesterone by cells in the ovary.

AFP. The levels of these substances are combined with mother's age to calculate the risk for Down's Syndrome. If the risk that the mother is carrying a fetus with Down's Syndrome is calculated to be more than 1 in 250, the mother is offered amniocentesis. In a small number of cases, the triple test indicates a high risk for other disorders, such as Edward's Syndrome (trisomy 18) or Turner's Syndrome, and this also leads to the offer of amniocentesis. In Down's Syndrome, the level of unconjugated estriol tends to be elevated and the level of AFP is low, whereas the levels of all three substances are low in Edwards's Syndrome. Abnormally high levels of AFP can indicate structural abnormalities such as neural-tube defects, as AFP "leaks" into the amniotic fluid from the fetus. At Addenbrooke's Hospital, roughly 60 percent of the amniotic-fluid samples analyzed come from mothers who first underwent the triple test screening. This is similar to the percentage reported here.

Late Maternal Age (25 Percent)

Some women decide to have an early amniocentesis, rather than first having the triple test. This is often due to late maternal age (over 35), which is associated with an elevated risk of Down's Syndrome. A number of mothers in this study said that they chose this direct route so as not to delay the amniocentesis, which would have become more emotionally difficult as the pregnancy progressed and, for example, the baby began to move. They saw their late age as a big enough risk factor, and did not wish to spend time on the triple test procedure.

Family History of Down's Syndrome (2.5 Percent)

These women underwent amniocentesis without triple screening, as they had family members with Down's Syndrome.

Maternal Anxiety (3.75 Percent)

These women underwent amniocentesis because of general anxiety about their pregnancies.

Scan (8.75 Percent)

A number of women underwent amniocentesis when scans revealed soft markers for Down's Syndrome or other conditions.

References

Abeliovich, D., Leiberman, J. R., Teuerstein, I., and Levy, J. 1984. Prenatal sex diagnosis: Testosterone and FSH levels in mid-trimester amniotic fluids. *Prenatal Diagnosis* 4: 347–353.

Aboitiz, F., Scheibel, A. B., and Zaidel, E. 1992. Morphometry of the sylvian fissure and the corpus callosum, with emphasis on sex differences. *Brain* 115, part 5: 1521–1541.

Abramovich, D. R. 1974. Human sexual differentiation—in utero influences. *Journal of Obstetrics and Gynecology* 81: 448–453.

Abramovich, D. R., Davidson, I. A., Longstaff, A., and Pearson, C. K. 1987. Sexual differentiation of the human midtrimester brain. *European Journal of Obstetrics, Gynecology, and Reproductive Biology* 25, no. 1: 7–14.

Abramovich, D. R., and Rowe, P. 1973. Foetal plasma testosterone levels at mid-pregnancy and at term: Relationship to foetal sex. *Journal of Endocrinology* 56: 621–622.

Adkins-Regan, E. 1999. Testosterone increases singing and aggression but not male-typical sexual partner preference in early estrogen treated zebra finches. *Hormones and Behavior* 35, no. 1: 63–70.

Ali, M., Balapure, A. K., Singh, D. R., Shukla, R. N., and Sahib, M. K. 1981). Ontogeny of alpha-foetoprotein in human foetal brain. *Brain Research* 207: 459–464.

Allen, L. S., Hines, M., Shryne, J. E., and Gorski, R. A. 1989. Two sexually dimorphic cell groups in the human brain. *Journal of Neuroscience* 9: 497–506.

Anderson, G. M., Horne, W. C., Chatterjee, D., and Cohen, D. J. 1990. The hyperserotonemia of autism. *Annals of New York Academy of Sciences* 600: 331–342.

Annett, M. 1967. The distribution of manual asymmetry. *British Journal of Psychology* 19: 327–333.

Annett, M. 1985. *Left, Right, Hand and Brain: The Right Shift Theory*. Erlbaum.

Annett, M. 1998. Handedness and cerebral dominance: The right shift theory. *Journal of Neuropsychiatry and Clinical Neuroscience* 10: 459–469.

Argyle, M., and Cook, M. 1976. *Gaze and Mutual Gaze*. Cambridge University Press.

Arnold, A. 1996. Genetically triggered sexual diffferentiation of brain and behaviour. *Hormones and Behavior* 30: 495–505.

Arnold, A. P. 1997. Sexual differentiation of the zebra finch song system: Positive evidence, negative evidence, null hypotheses and a paradigm shift. *Journal of Neurobiology* 33: 572–584.

Arnold, A. P., and Breedlove, S. M. 1985. Organizational and activational effects of sex steroids on brain and behavior: A reanalysis. *Hormones and Behavior* 19, no. 4: 469–498.

Arnold, A. P., and Gorski, R. A. 1984. Gonadal steroid induction of structural sex differences in the CNS. *Annual Review of Neurosciences* 7: 413–442.

Bachevalier, J., Hagger, C., and Bercu, B. 1989. Gender differences in visual habit formation in 3-month-old rhesus monkeys. *Developmental Psychobiology* 22, no. 6: 585–599.

Baker, S. W., and Ehrhardt, A. A. 1974. Prenatal androgen, intelligence and cognitive sex differences. In R. C. Friedman, R. M. Richart, and R. L. Van de Wiele, eds., *Sex Differences in Behaviour*. Wiley.

Bardin, C. W., and Catterall, J. F. 1981. Testosterone: A major determinant of extragenital sexual dimorphism. *Science* 211, no. 20: 1285–1294.

Baron-Cohen, S. 1989. Joint attention deficits in autism: Towards a cognitive analysis. *Development and Psychopathology* 1: 185–189.

Baron-Cohen, S. 1991. The theory of mind deficit in autism: How specific is it? *British Journal of Developmental Psychology* 9: 310–314.

Baron-Cohen, S. 1995. *Mindblindness: An Essay on Autism and Theory of Mind*. MIT Press.

Baron-Cohen, S. 1999. The extreme male-brain theory of autism. In H. Tager-Flusberg, ed., *Neurodevelopmental Disorders*. MIT Press.

Baron-Cohen, S. 2000. Autism: Deficits in folk psychology exist alongside superiority in folk physics. In S. Baron-Cohen, H. Tager-Flusberg, and D. Cohen, eds., *Understanding Other Minds*. Oxford University Press.

Baron-Cohen, S. 2002. The extreme male brain theory of autism. Trends in Cognitive Sciences 6: 248–254.

Baron-Cohen, S. 2003. *The Essential Difference: Men, Women, and the Extreme Male Brain*. Penguin/Perseus.

Baron-Cohen, S., and Hammer, J. 1997. Is autism an extreme form of the "male brain"? *Advances in Infancy Research* 2: 193–217.

Baron-Cohen, S., Jolliffe, T., Mortimore, C., and Robertson, M. 1997. Another advanced test of theory of mind: Evidence from very high functioning adults with autism or Asperger Syndrome. *Journal of Child Psychology and Psychiatry* 38, no. 7: 813–822.

Baron-Cohen, S., Spitz, A., and Cross, P. 1993. Can children with autism recognize surprise? *Cognition and Emotion* 7: 507–516.

Baron-Cohen, S., Wheelwright, S., Hill, J., Raste, Y., and Plumb, I. 2001. The "Reading the Mind in the eyes" test revised version: A study with normal adults, and adults with Asperger Syndrome or high-functioning autism. *Journal of Child Psychiatry and Psychiatry* 42: 241–252.

Bartsch, K., and Wellman, H. 1995. *Children Talk about the Mind*. Oxford University Press.

Bear, D., Schiff, D., Saver, J., Greenberg, M., and Freeman, R. 1986. Quantitative analysis of cerebral asymmetries. *Archives of Neurology* 43: 598–603.

Benenson, J. F. 1993. Greater preference among females than males for dyadic interaction in early childhood. *Child Development* 64, no. 2: 544–555.

Berenbaum, S. A., and Denburg, S. D. 1995. evaluating the empirical support for the role of testosterone in the Geschwind-Behan-

Galaburda model of cerebral lateralisation: Commentary on Bryden, McManus, and Bulman-Fleming. *Brain and Cognition* 27: 79–83.

Beyer, C. 1999. Estrogen and the developing mammalian brain. *Anatomy and Embryology* 199: 379–390.

Bidlingmaier, F., Strom, T. M., Dorr, H. G., Eisenmenger, W., and Knorr, D. 1987. Estrone and estradiol concentrations in human ovaries, testes, and adrenals during the first two years of life. *Journal of Clinical Endocrinology and Metabolism* 65, no. 5: 862–867.

Bidlingmaier, F., Versmold, H., and Knorr, D. 1974. Plasma oestrogens in newborns and infants. In M. Forest and J. Bertrand, eds., *Sexual Endocrinology of the Perinatal Period*. Paris: Institut National de la Sante et de la Recherche Medicale.

Biegon, A. 1990. Effects of steroid hormones on the serotonergic system. *Annals of New York Academy of Sciences* 600: 427–434.

Bishop, D. 1998. Development of the Children's Communicative Checklist (CCC): A method for assessing qualitative aspects of communicative impairment in children. *Journal of Child Psychology and Psychiatry* 39: 879–892.

Bixo, M., Backstrom, T., Winblad, B., and Andersson, A. 1995. Estradiol and testosterone in specific regions of the human female brain in different endocrine states. *Journal of Steroid Biochemistry and Molecular Biology* 55, no. 3–4: 297–303.

Bolton, P., Macdonald, H., Pickles, A., Rios, P., Goode, S., Crowson, M., Bailey, A., and Le Couteur, A. 1994. A case-control family history study of autism. *Journal of Child Psychology and Psychiatry* 35, no. 5: 877–900.

Breedlove, S. 1994. Sexual differentiation of the human nervous system. *Annual Review of Psychology* 45: 398–418.

Bregman, J. D., Dykens, E., Watson, M., Ort, S. I., and Leckman, J. F. 1987. Fragile X syndrome: Variability of phenotypic expression. *Journal of the American Academy of Child and Adolescent Psychiatry* 26: 463–471.

Brothers, L., Ring, B., and Kling, A. 1990. Responses of neurons in the macaque amygdala to complex social stimuli. *Behavioural Brain Research* 41: 199–213.

Brown, R., Hobson, P., Lee, A., and Stevenson, J. 1997. Are there "autistic-like" features in congenitally blind children? *Journal of Child Psychology and Psychiatry* 38: 693–704.

Bryden, M. P., McManus, I. C., and Bulman-Fleming, M. B. 1994. Evaluating the empirical support for the Geschwind-Behan-Galaburda model of cerebral lateralization. *Brain and Cognition* 26: 103–167.

Campbell, R., Heywood, C., Cowey, A., Regard, M., and Landis, T. 1990. Sensitivity to eye gaze in prosopagnosic patients and monkeys with superior temporal sulcus ablation. *Neuropsychologia* 28: 1123–1142.

Caviness, V. S., Kennedy, D. N., Richelme, C., Rademacher, J., and Filipek, P. A. 1996. The human brain age 7–11 years: A volumetric analysis based on magnetic resonance images. *Cerebral Cortex* 6: 726–736.

Chara, T. 1982. Proteins of the human placenta: Some general concepts. In J. G. Grudzinski and M. Seppala, eds., *Pregnancy Proteins*. Academic Press.

Christiansen, K., and Knussmann, R. 1987a. Androgen levels and components of aggressive behaviour in men. *Hormones and Behavior* 21, no. 2: 170–180.

Christiansen, K., and Knussmann, R. 1987b. Sex hormones and cognitive functioning in men. *Neuropsychobiology* 18, no. 1: 27–36.

Clark, M. M., Robertson, R. K., and Galef, B. G. 1996. Effects of perinatal testosterone on handedness of gerbils: Support for part of the Geschwind-Galaburda hypothesis. *Behavioral Neuroscience* 110, no. 2: 413–417.

Clark, M. M., Robertson, R. K., and Galef, B. G. 1993. Intrauterine position effects on sexually dimorphic asymmetries of Mongolian gerbils: Testosterone, eye-opening and handedness. *Developmental Psychobiology* 26: 185–194.

Cole-Harding, S., Mostad, A. L., and Wilson, J. R. 1988. Spatial ability in members of opposite-sex twin pairs. *Behavior Genetics* 18: 710.

Collaer, M. L., and Hines, M. 1995. Human behavioural sex differences: A role for gonadal hormones during early development? *Psychological Bulletin* 118, no. 1: 55–107.

Connellan, J., Baron-Cohen, S., Wheelwright, S., Ba'tki, A., and Ahluwalia, J. 2001. Sex differences in human neonatal social perception. *Infant Behavior and Development* 23: 113–118.

Corballis, M. C., and Morgan, M. J. 1978. On the biological basis of human laterality. *Behavioral and Brain Sciences* 2: 261–336.

Courchesne, E. 1997. Brainstem, cerebellar and limbic neuroanatomical abnormalities in autism. *Cognitive Neuroscience* 7: 269–278.

Creswell, C. S., and Skuse, D. H. 1999. Autism in association with Turner Syndrome: Genetic implications for male vulnerability to pervasive developmental disorders. *Neurocase* 5: 511–518.

Crucian, G. P., and Berenbaum, S. A. 1998. Sex differences in right hemisphere tasks. *Brain and Cognition* 36, no. 3: 377–389.

Davies, R. H., Harris, B., Thomas, D. R., Cook, N., Read, G., and Riad-Fahmy, D. 1992. Salivary testosterone levels and major depressive illness in men. *British Journal of Psychiatry* 161: 629–632.

Dawood, M. Y., and Saxena, B. B. 1977. Testosterone and dihydrotestosterone in maternal and cord blood and in amniotic fluid. *American Journal of Obstetrics and Gynecology* 129: 37–42.

de Courten-Myers, G. M. 1999. The human cerebral cortex: Gender differences in structure and function. *Journal of Neuropathology and Experimental Neurology* 58, no. 3: 217–226.

De Lacoste-Utamsing, C., and Holloway, R. L. 1982. Sexual dimorphism in the human corpus callosum. *Science* 216: 1431–1432.

De Vries, G., Rissman, E., Simerley, R, Yang, L., Scordalakes, E, Auger, C., Swain, A., Lovell-Badge, R., Burgoyne, P., and Arnold, A. 2002. A model system for study of sex chromosome effects on sexually dimorphic neural and behavioural traits. *Journal of Neuroscience* 2220: 9005–9014.

Dittman, R. W., Kappes, M. H., and Kappes, M. E. 1992. Sexual behaviour in adult and adolescent females with congenital adrenal hyperplasia. *Psychoneuroendocrinology* 17: 153–170.

Dittman, R. W., Kappes, M. H., Kappes, M. E., Borger, D., Stegner, H., Willig, R. H., and Wallis, H. 1990. Congenital adrenal hyperplasia I: Gender related behaviour and attitudes in female patients and sisters. *Psychoneuroendocrinology* 15: 401–420.

Dollaghan, C. A., Campbell, T. F., Paradise, J. L., Feldman, H. M., Janosky, J. E., Pitcairn, D. N., and Kurs-Lasky, M. 1999. Maternal education and measures of early speech and language. *Journal of Speech, Language, and Hearing Research* 42, no. 6: 1432–1443.

Donahoe, P. K., Cate, R. L., and MacLaughlin, D. T. 1987. Mullerian inhibitory substance: Gene structure and action of a foetal regressor. *Recent Progress in Hormone Research* 43: 431–468.

Dörner, G. 1976. Hormones and Brain Differentiation. Elsevier.

Dörner, G. 1978. Hormones, brain development and fundamental processes of life. In G. Dörner and M. Kawakami, eds., *Hormones and Brain Development*. Elsevier/North-Holland Biomedical Press.

Dörner, G., Docke, F., Gotz, F., Rohde, W., Stahl, F., and Tonjes, R. 1987. Sexual differentiation of gonadotropin secretion, sexual orientation and gender role behaviour. *Journal of Steroid Biochemistry* 27, no. 4–6: 1081–1087.

Dörner, G., Schenk, B., Schmiedel, B., and Ahrens, L. 1983. Stressful events in prenatal life of bi- and homosexual men. *Experimental Clinical Endocrinology* 81: 83–87.

Elkadi, S., Nicholls, M. E., and Clode, D. 1999. Handedness in opposite and same-sex dizygotic twins: Testing and testosterone hypothesis. *Neuroreport* 10, no. 2: 333–336.

Fenson, L., Dale, P., Reznick, J., Thal, D., Bates, E., Hartung, J, Pethick, S., and Reilly, J. 1993. MacArthur Communicative Development Inventory: Users Guide and technical manual. Singular.

Fenson, L., Dale, P. S., Reznick, J. S., Bates, E., Thal, D. J., and Pethick, S. J. 1994. Variability in early communicative development. *Monographs of the Society for Research in Child Development* 59, no. 5.

Finegan, J. A., Sitarenios, G., Bolan, P. L., and Sarabura, A. D. 1996. Children whose mothers had second trimester amniocentesis: Follow up at school age. *British Journal of Obstetrics and Gynaecology* 103, no. 3: 214–218.

Finegan, J. K., Bartleman, B., and Wong, P. Y. 1991. A window for the study of prenatal sex hormone influences on postnatal development. *Journal of Genetic Psychology* 150, no. 1: 101–112.

Finegan, J. K., Niccols, G. A., and Sitarenios, G. 1992. Relations between prenatal testosterone levels and cognitive abilities at 4 years. *Developmental Psychology* 28, no. 6: 1075–1089.

Fitch, R., and Denenberg, V. 1998. A role for ovarian hormones in sexual differentiation of the brain. *Behavioural and Brain Sciences* 21: 311–352.

Fitch, R., Cowell, P. E., Schrott, L. M., and Denenberg, V. H. 1991. Corpus callosum: Ovarian hormones and feminization. *Brain Research* 542, no. 2: 313–317.

Flavell, J., Green, F., Herrera, C., and Flavell, E. 1991. Young children's knowledge about visual perception: Lines of sight must be straight. *British Journal of Developmental Psychology* 9: 73–87.

Fuchs, F., and Klopper, A. 1983. *Endocrinology of Pregnancy*. Harper and Row.

Gazzaniga, M. S., Ivry, R. B., and Mangun, G. R. 1998. *Cognitive Neuroscience: The Biology of the Mind*. Norton.

Geary, D. C. 1996. Sexual selection and sex differences in mathematical abilities. *Behavioral and Brain Sciences* 19: 229–284.

Geary, D. 1998. *Male, Female: The Evolution of Human Sex Differences*. American Psychological Association.

George, F. W., and Wilson, J. D. 1992. Embryology of the genital tract. In P. C. Walsh, A. B. Retik, and T. A. Stamey, eds., *Campbell's Urology*, sixth edition. Saunders.

Geschwind, N., and Behan, P. 1982. Left-handedness: Association with immune disease, migraine and developmental learning disorder. *Proceedings of the National Academy of Sciences (USA)* 79: 5097–5100.

Geschwind, N., and Galaburda, A. M. 1985a. Cerebral lateralisation: Biological mechanisms, associations and pathology: I. A hypothesis and a program for research. *Archives of Neurology* 42: 428–459.

Geschwind, N., and Galaburda, A. M. 1985b. Cerebral lateralisation: Biological mechanisms, associations and pathology: II. A hypothesis and a program for research. *Archives of Neurology* 42: 521–552.

Geschwind, N., and Galaburda, A. M. 1985c. Cerebral lateralisation: Biological mechanisms, associations and pathology: III. A hypothesis and a program for research. *Archives of Neurology* 42: 634–654.

Gillberg, C., Rasmussen, P., and Wahlstrom, J. 1982. Long-term follow-up of children born after amniocentesis. *Clinical Genetics* 21, no. 1: 69–73.

Gillberg, C., and Wing, L. 1999. Autism: Not an extremely rare disorder. *Acta Psychiatrica Scandinavica* 99, no. 6: 399–406.

Gitlin, D., Pericelli, A., and Gitlin, G. M. 1972. Synthesis of alphafetoprotein by liver, yolk sac and gastrointestinal tract of the human conceptus. *Cancer Research* 32: 979–982.

Goldman, S., and Nottebohm, F. 1983. Neuronal production, migration and differentiation in a vocal control nucleus of the adult female canary brain. *Proceedings of the National Academy of Sciences (USA)* 80: 2390.

Gouchie, C., and Kimura, D. 1991. The relationship between testosterone levels and cognitive ability patterns. *Psychoneuroendocrinology* 16, no. 4: 323–334.

Goy, R. W., Bercovitch, F. B., and McBrair, M. C. 1988. Behavioural masculinization is independent of genital masculinization in prenatally androgenized female rhesus macaques. *Hormones and Behavior* 22, no. 4: 552–571.

Goy, R. W., and McEwen, B. S. 1980. *Sexual Differentiation of the Brain*. MIT Press.

Grimshaw, G. M., Bryden, M. P., and Finegan, J. K. 1995a. Relations between prenatal testosterone and cerebral lateralisation in children. *Neuropsychology* 9, no. 1: 68–79.

Grimshaw, G. M., Sitarenios, G., and Finegan, J. K. 1995b. Mental rotation at 7 years: relations with prenatal testosterone levels and spatial play experiences. *Brain and Cognition* 29: 85–100.

Grumbach, M. M., and Conte, F. A. 1992. Disorders of sex differentiation. In *Williams Textbook of Endocrinology*. Saunders.

Gurney, M. E., and Konishi, M. 1980. Hormone-induced sexual differentiation of brain and behaviour in zebra finches. *Science* 208: 1380–1383.

Hadley, M. E. 2000. *Endocrinology*. Prentice-Hall.

Halpern, D. 1992. *Sex Differences in Cognitive Ability*. Erlbaum.

Hampson, E. 1990. Estrogen related variations in human spatial and articulatory-motor skills. *Psychoneuroendocrinology* 15: 97–111.

Hampson, E., and Kimura, D. 1988. Reciprocal effects of hormonal fluctuations on human motor and perceptual-spatial skills. *Behavioral Neuroscience* 102, no. 3: 456–459.

Hampson, E., and Moffat, S. D. 1994. Is testosterone related to spatial cognition and hand preference in humans? *Brain and Cognition* 26: 255–266.

Hampson, E., Rovet, J. F., and Altmann, D. 1994. Spatial reasoning in children with congenital adrenal hyperplasia due to 21-hydroxylase deficiency. Presented at meeting of International Society of Psychoneuroendocrinology, Seattle.

Harris, G. W., and Levine, S. 1962. Sexual differentiation of the brain and its experimental control. *Journal of Physiology* 181: 379–400.

Hauser, H., and Gandelman, R. 1983. Contiguity to males in utero affects avoidance responding in adult female mice. *Science* 220, no. 4595: 437–438.

Hay, D. F. 1980. Multiple functions of proximity seeking in infancy. *Child Development* 51, no. 3: 636–645.

Helleday, J., Siwers, B., Ritzen, E. M., and Hugdahl, K. 1994. Normal lateralization for handedness and ear advantage in a verbal dichotic listening task in women with congenital adrenal hyperplasia (CAH). *Neuropsychologia* 32: 875–880.

Henderson, B. A., and Berenbaum, S. A. 1997. Sex-typed play in opposite-sex twins. *Developmental Psychobiology* 31, no. 2: 115–123.

Hermle, L., and Oepen, G. 1987. Hemispheric laterality and childhood autism. *Nervenarzt* 60: 370.

Hier, D. B., and Crowley, W. F. 1982. Spatial ability in androgen-deficient men. *New England Journal of Medicine* 306: 1202–1205.

Hines, M., and Shipley, C. 1984. Prenatal exposure to diethylstilbestrol (des) and the development of sexually dimorphic cognitive abilities and cerebral lateralisation. *Developmental Psychology* 20, no. 1: 81–94.

Hiscock, M., Inch, R., Jacek, C., Hiscock-Kalil, C., and Kalil, K. M. 1993. Is there a sex difference in human laterality? An exhaustive survey of auditory laterality studies from six neuropsychology journals. *Journal of Clinical and Experimental Neuropsychology* 16, no. 3: 423–435.

Hobson, R. P. 1993. *Autism and the Development of the Mind*. Erlbaum.

Holloway, R. L., Anderson, P. J., Defendini, R., and Harper, C. 1993. Sexual dimorphism of the human corpus callosum from three independent samples: relative size of the corpus callosum. *American Journal of Physical Anthropology* 92, no. 4: 481–498.

Hoon, A., and Reiss, A. 1992. The mesial-temporal lobe and autism: Case report and review. *Developmental Medicine and Child Neurology* 34: 253–259.

Huttenlocher, J., Haight, W., Bryk, A., Seltzer, M., and Lyons, T. 1991. Early language growth: Relation to language input and gender. *Developmental Psychology* 27: 236–248.

Hyde, J. S., and Linn, M. C. 1988. Gender differences in verbal ability: A meta-analysis. *Psychological Bulletin* 104: 53–69.

Imperato-McGinley, J., Pichardo, M., Gautier, T., Voyer, D., and Bryden, M. P. 1991. Cognitive abilities in androgen-insensitive subjects: Comparison with control males and females from the same kindred. *Clinical Endocrinology* 34, no. 5: 341–347.

Insel, T. R. 1992. Oxytocin—a neuropeptide for affiliation: Evidence from behavioural, receptor autoradiographic and comparative studies. *Psychoneuroendocrinology* 17, no. 1: 3–35.

Insel, T. 1997. A neurobiological basis of social attachment. *American Journal of Psychiatry* 154: 726–735.

Insel, T. R., O'Brien, D. J., and Leckman, J. F. 1999. Oxytocin, vasopressin, and autism: Is there a connection? *Biological Psychiatry* 45: 145–157.

Jacklin, C. N., Maccoby, E. E., and Doering, C. H. 1983. Neonatal sex-steroid hormones and timidity in 6–18-month-old boys and girls. *Developmental Psychobiology* 16, no. 3: 163–168.

Jacklin, C. N., Wilcox, K. T., and Maccoby, E. E. 1988. Neonatal sex-steroid hormones and cognitive abilities at six years. *Developmental Psychobiology* 21, no. 6: 567–574.

James, W. H. 1983. Timing of fertilization and the sex ratio of offspring. In N. G. Bennett, ed., *Sex Selection of Children*. Academic Press.

James, W. H. 1986. Hormonal control of sex ratio. *Journal of Theoretical Biology* 118: 427–441.

Jarrold, C., Jimenez, F., and Butler, D. 1998. Evidence for a Link between Weak Central Coherence and Theory of Mind Deficits in Autism. Paper presented at annual conference of British Psychological Society, Developmental Section, Lancaster.

Jolliffe, T., and Baron-Cohen, S. 1997. Are people with autism and asperger syndrome faster than normal on the embedded figures test? *Journal of Child Psychology and Psychiatry* 38, no. 5: 527–534.

Jost, A. 1961. The role of foetal hormones in prenatal development. *Harvey Lectures* 55: 201–226.

Jost, A. 1972. A new look at the mechanism controlling sexual differentiation in mammals. *Johns Hopkins Medical Journal* 130: 38–53.

Kandel, D. B., and Udry, J. R. 1999. Prenatal effects of maternal smoking on daughters' smoking: Nicotine or testosterone exposure? *American Journal of Public Health* 89, no. 9: 1377–1383.

Kawashima, R., Sugiura, M., Kato, T., Nakamura, A., Hatano, K., Ito, K., Fukuda, H., Kojima, S., and Nakamura, K. 1999. The human amygdala plays an important role in gaze monitoring. *Brain* 122: 779–783.

Kertesz, A., Polk, M., Howell, J., and Black, S. E. 1987. Cerebral dominance, sex, and callosal size in MRI. *Neurology* 37: 1385–1388.

Kimura, D. 1999. *Sex and Cognition.* MIT Press.

Kimura, D., and Hampson, E. 1994. Cognitive pattern in men and women is influenced by fluctuations in sex hormones. *Current Directions in Psychological Science* 3: 57–61.

Kimura, D., and Toussaint, C. 1991. Sex differences in cognitive function vary with the season. *Society for Neuroscience Abstracts* 17: 868.

Kleinke, C. 1986. Gaze and eye contact: A research review. *Psychological Bulletin* 100: 78–100.

Knecht, S., Deppe, M., Drager, B., Bobe, L., Lohmann, H., Ringelstein, E., and Hennigsen, H. 2000. Language lateralisation in healthy right-handers. *Brain* 123: 74–81.

Knickmeyer, R., Baron-Cohen, S., Raggatt, P., and Taylor, K. In press. Foetal testosterone, social cognition, and restricted interests in children. *Journal of Child Psychology and Psychiatry*.

Knussmann, R., Christiansen, K., and Couwenbergs, C. 1986. Relations between sex hormone levels and sexual behaviour in men. *Archives of Sex Behavior* 15, no. 5: 429–445.

Kreuz, L. E., Rose, R. M., and Jennings, J. R. 1972. Suppression of plasma testosterone levels and psychological stress. *Archives of Genetic Psychiatry* 26: 479–482.

Langdell, T. 1978. Recognition of faces: An approach to the study of autism. *Journal of Child Psychology and Psychiatry* 19: 225–238.

Lansdell, H., and Davie, J. C. 1972. Massa intermedia: Possible relation to intelligence. *Neuropsychologia* 10: 207–210.

LeMay, M., and Culebras, A. 1972. Human brain: Morphologic differences in the hemispheres demonstrable by carotid ateriography. *New England Journal of Medicine* 287: 168–170.

Levy, J. 1976. Possible basis of the evolution of lateral specialisation of the human brain. *Nature* 224: 614–615.

Linn, M. C., and Petersen, A. C. 1985. Emergence and characterisation of sex differences in spatial ability: A meta-analysis. *Child Development* 56: 1479–1498.

Lord, C. 1995. Follow-up of two-year-olds referred for possible autism. *Journal of Child Psychology and Psychiatry* 36, no. 8: 1365–1382.

Lord, C., and Schopler, E. 1987. Neurobiological Implications of Sex Differences in Autism. In E. Schopler and G. B. Mesibov, eds., *Neurobiological Issues in Autism*. Plenum.

Lutchmaya, S., and Baron-Cohen, S. 2002. Human sex differences in social and non-social looking preferences at 12 months of age. *Infant Behaviour and Development* 25: 319–325.

Lutchmaya, S., Baron-Cohen, S., and Raggatt, P. 2002. Foetal testosterone and vocabulary size in 18- and 24-month-old infants. *Infant Behavior and Development* 24, no. 4: 418–424.

Lutchmaya, S., Baron-Cohen, S., Raggatt, P., and Manning, J. In press. Maternal 2nd to 4th digit ratios and foetal testosterone. *Cortex*.

Lutchmaya, S., Baron-Cohen, S., and Raggett, P. 2002. Foetal testosterone and eye contact in 12 month old infants. *Infant Behavior and Development* 25: 327–335.

Maccoby, E. 1990. Gender and relationships: A developmental account. *American Psychologist* 45: 513–520.

Maccoby, E. E., Doering, C. H., Jacklin, C. N., and Kraemer, H. 1979. Concentrations of sex hormones in umbilical cord blood: Their relation to sex and birth order of infants. *Child Development* 50: 632–642.

Maccoby, E. E., and Jacklin, C. N. 1974. *The Psychology of Sex Differences*. Stanford University Press.

Mack, C. M., McGivern, R. F., Hyde, L. A., and Denenberg, V. H. 1996. Absence of postnatal testosterone fails to demasculinise the male rat's corpus callosum. *Developmental Brain Research* 95, no. 2: 252–255.

Mackenberg, E. J., Broverman, D. M., Vogel, W., and Klaiber, E. L. 1974. Morning-to-afternoon changes in cognitive performances and in the electroencephalogram. *Journal of Educational Psychology* 66: 238–246.

MacLusky, N. J., and Naftolin, F. 1981. Sexual differentiation of the central nervous system. *Science* 211: 1294–1303.

Mann, D. R., Gould, K. G., and Collins, D. C. 1989. Blockade of neonatal activation of the pituitary-testicular axis: effect on peripubertal luteinizing hormone and testosterone secretion and on testicular development in male monkeys. *Journal of Clinical Endocrinology and Metabolism* 68: 600–607.

Mansukhani, V., Adkins-Regan, E., and Yang, S. 1996. Sexual partner preference in female zebra finches: The role of early hormones and social environment. *Hormones and Behavior* 30, no. 4: 506–513.

Martin, C. R. 1985. *Endocrine Physiology*. Oxford University Press.

Matuszczyk, J. V., and Larsson, K. 1995. Sexual preference and feminine and masculine sexual behaviour of male rats prenatally exposed to antiandrogen or antiestrogen. *Hormones and Behavior* 29, no. 2: 191–206.

Maurer, D., and Salapatek, P. 1976. Developmental changes in the scanning of faces by young infants. *Child Development* 47: 523–527.

McBride, P. A., Anderson, G. M., Hertzig, M. E., Sweeney, J. A., Kream, J., Cohen, D. J., and Mann, J. J. 1989. Serotonergic responsivity in male young adults with autistic disorder. *Archives of General Psychiatry* 46: 213–221.

McEwen, B. S. 1994. How do sex and stress hormones affect nerve cells? *Annals of New York Academy of Sciences* 14 (743): 1–16.

McGlone, J. 1980. Sex differences in human brain asymmetry: A critical survey. *Behavioral and Brain Sciences* 3: 215–263.

McManus, I. C., and Bryden, M. P. 1991. Geschwind's theory of cerebral lateralisation: Developing a formal, causal model. *Psychological Bulletin* 110, no. 2: 237–253.

Meaney, M., and McEwen. 1986. Testosterone implants into the amygdala during the neonatal period masculinise the social play of juvenile female rats. *Brain Research* 398: 324–328.

Meaney, M. J., Aitken, D. H., Jensen, L. K., McGinnis, M. Y., and McEwen, B. S. 1985. Nuclear and cytosolic androgen receptor levels in the limbic brain of neonatal male and female rats. *Brain Research* 355, no. 2: 179–185.

Michael, R. P., Rees, H. D., and Bonsall, R. W. 1989. Sites in the male primate brain at which testosterone acts as an androgen. *Brain Research* 502, no. 1: 11–20.

Miller, G. 2000. *The Mating Mind.* Heinemann.

Mirenda, P., Donnellan, A., and Yoder, D. 1983. Gaze behaviour: A new look at an old problem. *Journal of Autism and Developmental Disorders* 13: 397–409.

Modahl, C., Green, L., Fein, D., Morris, M., Waterhouse, L., Feinstin, C., and Levin, H. 1998. Plasma oxytocin levels in autistic children. *Biological Psychiatry* 43: 270–277.

Moffat, S. D., and Hampson, E. 1996. A curvilinear relationship between testosterone and spatial cognition in humans: Possible influences of hand preference. *Psychoneuroendocrinology* 21, no. 3: 323–337.

Moffat, S. D., Hampson, E., Wickett, J. C., Vernon, P. A., and Lee, D. H. 1997. Testosterone is correlated with regional morphology of the human corpus callosum. *Brain Research* 767, no. 2: 297–304.

Murphy, J., and Greer, M. 1986. The human medial amygdaloid nucleus: No evidence for sex difference in volume. *Brain Research* 365: 321–324.

Nagamani, M., McDonough, P. G., Ellegood, J. O., and Mahesh, V. B. 1979. Maternal and amniotic fluid steroids throughout human pregnancy. *American Journal of Obstetrics and Gynecology* 134, no. 6: 674.

Nass, R., Baker, S., Speiser, P., Virdis, R., Balsamo, A., Cacciari, E., Loche, A., Dumic, M., and New, M. 1987. Left-hand bias in female congenital adrenal hyperplasia patients. *Neurology* 37: 711–715.

New, M. I., and Levine, L. S. 1984. Steroid 21-hydroxylase deficiency. In M. I. New and L. S. Levine, eds., *Adrenal Diseases in Childhood*. Karger.

Nicholls, M. E. R., and Forbes, S. 1996. Handedness and its association with gender-related psychological and physiological characteristics. *Journal of Clinical and Experimental Neuropsychology* 118, no. 6: 905–910.

Nottebohm, F., and Arnold, A. P. 1976. Sexual dimorphism in vocal control areas of the songbird brain. *Science* 194: 211–213.

Nunez, J. L., and Juraska, J. M. 1998. The size of the splenium of the rat corpus callosum: Influence of hormones, sex ratio, and neonatal cryoanesthesia. *Developmental Psychobiology* 33, no. 4: 295–303.

Obrzut, J. E. 1994. The Geschwind-Behan-Galaburda theory of cerebral lateralisation: Thesis, antithesis and synthesis? *Brain and Cognition* 26: 267–274.

O'Callaghan, M. J., Tudehope, D. I., Dugdale, A. E., Mohay, H., Burns, Y., and Cook, F. 1987. Handedness in children with birthweight below 1000 g. *Lancet* 1, no. 8542: 1155.

Pakkenberg, H., and Gundersen, H. J. 1997. Neocortical neuron numbers in humans: Effect of sex and age. *Journal of Comparative Neurology* 384: 312–320.

Pakkenberg, H., and Voigt, J. 1964. Brain weight of the Danes. *Acta Anatomica (Basel)* 56, no. 4: 297–307.

Perrett, D., Harries, M., Mistlin, A., Hietanen, J., Benson, P., Bevan, R., Thomas, S., Oram, M., Ortega, J., and Brierley, K. 1990. Social signals analyzed at the single cell level: Someone is looking at me, something touched me, something moved! *International Journal of Comparative Psychology* 4: 25–55.

Perrett, D., Smith, P., Potter, D., Mistlin, A., Head, A., Milner, A., and Jeeves, M. 1985. Visual cells in the temporal cortex sensitive to face view and gaze direction. *Proceedings of the Royal Society of London* B223: 293–317.

Phillips, W., Baron-Cohen, S., and Rutter, M. 1992. The role of eye-contact in the detection of goals: Evidence from normal toddlers, and

children with autism or mental handicap. *Development and Psychopathology* 4: 375–383.

Plante, E., Boliek, C., Binkiewicz, A., and Erly, W. K. 1996. Elevated androgen, brain development and language/learning disabilities in children with congenital adrenal hyperplasia. *Developmental Medicine and Child Neurology* 38: 423–437.

Podrouzek, W., and Furrow, D. 1988. Preschoolers' use of eye contact while speaking—the influence of sex, age and conversational partner. *Journal of Psycholinguistic Research* 17, no. 2: 89–98.

Purifoy, F. E., and Koopmans, L. H. 1979. Androstenedione, testosterone and free testosterone concentrations in women of various occupations. *Social Biology* 26: 179–188.

Reinisch, J. M., and Sanders, S. A. 1992. Effects of prenatal exposure to diethylstilboestrol (DES) on hemispheric laterality and spatial ability in human males. *Hormones and Behavior* 26, no. 1: 62–75.

Repe, G. J., and Albrecht, E. D. 1990. Actions of placental and foetal adrenal steroid hormones in primate pregnancy. *Endocrine Review* 11: 124–150.

Reynell, J., and Huntley, M. 1985. *Reynell Development Language Scales*, second revision. NFER-Nelson.

Ridley, M. 1993. *The Red Queen*. Penguin.

Robinson, J., Judd, H., Young, P., Jones, D., and Yen, S. 1977. Amniotic fluid androgens and estrogens in midgestation. *Journal of Clinical Endocrinology* 45: 755–761.

Rodeck, C. H., Gill, D., Rosenberg, D. A., and Collins, W. P. 1985. Testosterone levels in midtrimester maternal and foetal plasma and amniotic fluid. Prenat Diag 5, no. 3: 175–181.

Roof, R. L., and Havens, M. D. 1992. Testosterone improves maze performance and induces development of a male hippocampus in females. *Brain Research* 572, no. 1–2: 310–313.

Rose, N. R., and Mackay, I. R. 1985. Genetic predisposition to autoimmune diseases. In N. R. Rose and I. R. Mackay, eds., *The Autoimmune Diseases*. Academic Press.

Rubin, R. T. 1981. Sex steroid hormone dynamics in endogenous depression: A review. *International Journal of Mental Health* 10: 43–59.

Rubinow, D. R., and Schmidt, P. J. 1996. Androgens, brain, and behaviour. *American Journal of Psychiatry* 153, no. 8: 974–984.

Saal, F. S., Vom, Grant, W. M., McMullen, C. W., and Laves, K. S. 1983. High fetal estrogen concentrations: Correlation with increased adult sexual activity and decreased aggression in male mice. *Science* 220: 1306–1308.

Saltvedt, S., and Almstrom, H. 1999. Fetal loss rate after second trimester amniocentesis at different gestational age. *Acta Obstetrica Gynecolica Scandinavica* 78, no. 1: 1–3.

Schafer, G., and Plunkett, K. 1998. Rapid word learning by fifteen-month-olds under tightly controlled conditions. *Child Development* 69, no. 2: 309–320.

Segalowitz, S. J., and Bryden, M. P. 1983. Individual differences in hemispheric representation of language. In S. J. Segalowitz, ed., *Language Functions and Brain Organization*. Academic Press.

Servin, A., Bohlin, G., and Berlin, L. 1999. Sex differences in 1-, 3- and 5-year-olds' toy-choice in a structured play session. *Scandinavian Journal of Psychology* 40: 43–48.

Shah, A., and Frith, U. 1983. An islet of ability in autistic children. *Journal of Child Psychology and Psychiatry* 24, no. 4: 613–620.

Shaywitz, S. E., Shaywitz, B. A., Fletcher, J. M., and Escobar, M. D. 1990. Prevalence of reading disability in boys and girls: Results of the Connecticut Longitudinal Study. *JAMA* 264, no. 8: 998–1002.

Sigman, M., Mundy, P., Sherman, T., and Ungerer, J. 1986. Social interactions of autistic, mentally retarded and normal children and their caregivers. *Journal of Child Psychology and Psychiatry* 27, no. 5: 647–656.

Simerly, R. B., Swanson, L. W., and Gorski, R. A. 1985. Adrenalcortical influence on rat brain tryptophan hydroxylase activity. *Brain Research* 340: 91–98.

Skuse, D. 2000. Imprinting, the X-chromosome, and the male brain: Explaining sex differences in the liability to autism. *Pediatric Research* 47, no. 1: 9–16.

Skuse, D. H., James, R. S., Bishop, D. V. M., Coppin, B., Dalton, P., Aamodt-Leeper, G., Bacarese-Hamilton, M., Creswell, C., McGurk, R., and Jacobs, P. A. 1997. Evidence from Turner's Syndrome of an

imprinted X-linked locus affecting cognitive function. *Nature* 387: 705–708.

Smail, P. J., Reyes, F. I., Winter, J. S. D., and Faiman, C. 1981. The fetal hormonal environment and its effect on the morphogenesis of the genital system. In S. J. Kogan and E. S. E. Hafez, eds., *Pediatric Andrology*. Martinus Nijhoff.

Stahl, F., Gotz, F., Poppe, I., Amendt, P., and Dörner, G. 1978. Pre- and early postnatal testosterone levels in rat and human. In G. Dörner and M. Kawakami, eds., *Hormones and Brain Development*. Elsevier.

Stern, D. 1977. *The First Relationship: Infant and Mother*. Open Books.

Stryer, L. 1995. *Biochemistry*, fourth edition. Freeman.

Swaab, D. F., and Fliers, E. 1985. A sexually dimorphic nucleus in the human brain. *Science* 228, no. 4703: 1112–1115.

Swaab, D. F., and Hofman, M. A. 1988. Sexual differentiation of the human hypothalamus: ontogeny of the sexually dimorphic nucleus of the preoptic area. *Developmental Brain Research* 44, no. 2: 314–318.

Swettenham, J., Baron-Cohen, S., Charman, T., Cox, A., Baird, G., Drew, A., Rees, L., and Wheelwright, S. 1998. The frequency and distribution of spontaneous attention shifts between social and nonsocial stimuli in autistic, typically developing, and non-autistic developmentally delayed infants. *Journal of Child Psychology and Psychiatry* 9: 747–753.

Tallal, P. 1991. Hormonal influences in developmental learning disabilities. *Psychoneuroendocrinology* 16, no. 1–3: 203–211.

Tallal, P., Ross, R., and Curtiss, S. 1989. Unexpected sex-ratios in families of language/learning-impaired children. *Neuropsychologia* 27, no. 2: 987–998.

Tordjman, S., Anderson, G. M., McBride, P. A., Hertzig, M. E., Snow, M. E., Hall, L. M., Ferrari, P., and Cohen, D. J. 1995. Plasma androgens in autism. *Journal of Autism and Developmental Disorders* 25, no. 3: 295–304.

Tordjman, S., and Ferrari, P. 1992. Testosterone in infantile autism. Presented at WAPID Fifth World Congress, Chicago.

Tordjman, S., Ferrari, P., Sulmont, V., Duyme, M., and Roubertoux, P. 1997. Androgenic activity in autism. *American Journal of Psychiatry* 154, no. 11: 1626–1627.

Trevarthen, C. 1979. Communication and cooperation in early infancy: A description of primary intersubjectivity. In M. Bullowa, ed., *Before Speech*. Cambridge University Press.

Trivers, R. L. and Willard, D. 1973. Natural selection of parental ability to vary the sex ratio of offspring. *Science* 179: 90–91.

Van Lith, J. M. M., Beekhuis, J. J., Van Loon, A. J., Mantingh, A., De Wolf, B. T. H. M., and Breed, A. S. P., M. 1991. Alpha-fetoprotein in fetal serum, amniotic fluid and maternal serum. *Prenatal Diagnosis* 11: 625–628.

Wada, J. A., Clarke, R., and Hamm, A. 1975. Cerebral hemispheric asymmetry in humans. *Archives of Neurology* 32: 239–246.

Ward, I. L. 1977. Exogenous androgen activates female behaviour in non-copulating, prenatally stressed male rats. *Physiological Psychology* 91: 465–471.

Wathen, N. C., Campbell, D. J., Kitau, M. J., and Chard, T. 1993. Alphafetoprotein levels in amniotic fluid in amniotic fluid from 8 to 18 weeks of pregnancy. *British Journal of Obstetrics and Gynaecology* 100: 380–382.

Weissman, M. M., Leaf, P. J., Tischler, G. L., Blazer, D. G., Karno, M., Bruce, M. L., and Florio, L. P. 1988. Affective disorders in five United States communities. *Psychological Medicine* 18, no. 1: 141–153.

Westney, L., Bruney, R., Ross, B., Clark, J. F., Rajguru, S., and Ahluwalia, B. 1991. Evidence that gonadal hormone levels in amniotic fluid are decreased in males born to alcohol users in humans. *Alcohol and Alcoholism* 26, no. 4: 403–407.

Wicker, B., Michel, F., Henaff, M., and Decety, J. 1998. Brain regions involved in the perception of gaze: A PET study. *Neuroimage* 8: 221–227.

Williams, C. L., Barnett, A. M., and Meck, W. H. 1990. Organizational effects of gonadal secretions on sexual differentiation in spatial memory. *Behavioral Neuroscience* 104: 84–97.

Wilson, J. D., Foster, D. W., Kronenberg, H. M., and Larsen, P. R. 1998. *Williams Textbook of Endocrinology*. Saunders.

Wing, L. 1981a. Asperger syndrome: a clinical account. *Psychological Medicine* 11: 115–130.

Wing, L. 1981b. Sex ratios in early childhood autism and related conditions. *Psychiatry Research* 5: 129–137.

Witelson, S. 1985. The brain connection: The corpus callosum is larger in left-handers. *Science* 229: 665–668.

Witelson, S. F. 1976. Sex and the single hemisphere: Specialisation of the right hemisphere for spatial processing. *Science* 193: 425–427.

Witelson, S. F. 1991. Neural sexual mosaicism: Sexual differentiation of the human temporo-parietal region for functional asymmetry. *Psychoneuroendocrinology* 16, no. 1–3: 131–153.

Witelson, S. F., and Goldsmith, C. H. 1991. The relationship of hand preference to anatomy of the corpus callosum in men. *Brain Research* 545 (1–2): 175–182.

Witelson, S. F., and Nowakowski, R. S. 1991. Left out axons make men right: a hypothesis for the origin of handedness and functional asymmetry. *Neuropsychologia* 29, no. 4: 327–333.

Young, A., Hellawell, D., De Wal, C., and Johnson, M. 1996. Facial expression processing after amygdalectomy. *Neuropsychologia* 34: 31–39.

Zaidel, E., Clarke, J. M., and Suyenobu, B. 1990. Hemispheric independence: A paradigm case for cognitive neuroscience. In A. B. Scheibel and A. F. Wechsler, eds., *Neurobiology of Higher Cognitive Function*. Guildford.

Zucker, K. J., Bradley, S. J., Oliver, G., Blake, J., Fleming, S., and Hood, J. 1996. Psychosexual development of women with congenital adrenal hyperplasia. *Hormones and Behavior* 30, no. 4: 300–318.

Index

Printed in the United States
by Baker & Taylor Publisher Services

Printed in the United States
by Baker & Taylor Publisher Services